Obstetrics for Anaesth

Dedications

John Clift
To my wife Katie, who had the original idea for this book

Alexander Heazell
To my Mother and Father, for their support and encouragement

Contents

Contributors

Julian Chilvers MBChB FRCA
Consultant Anaesthetist
City Hospital
Sandwell and West Birmingham
    Hospitals NHS Trust
Birmingham, UK

Wilson T F Chimbira MBChB, DA (UZ).
    FRCA (UK)
Lecturer in Anaesthesiology
University of Michigan
Ann Arbor
Michigan, USA

John Clift MBChB FRCA
Consultant Anaesthetist
City Hospital
Sandwell and West Birmingham
    Hospitals NHS Trust
Birmingham, UK

Katie Clift MBChB MRCS FRCA
Specialist Registrar in Anaesthetics and
    Intensive Care
City Hospital
Sandwell and West Birmingham
    Hospitals NHS Trust
Birmingham, UK

Paul Dias BMedSci (Hons) BMBS
    MRCP (UK)
Specialist Registrar in Anaesthetics and
    Intensive Care
Royal Wolverhampton Hospitals NHS
    Trust
Wolverhampton, UK

Joanna Gillham MD MRCOG
Consultant in
    Feto-Maternal Medicine
St Mary's Hospital
Manchester, UK

Alexander Heazell MBChB
Clinical Research Fellow
Maternal and Fetal Health
    Research Centre
St Mary's Hospital and University of
    Manchester
Manchester, UK

Jenny Myers MBBS PhD MRCOG
Clinical Lecturer
Maternal and Fetal Health Research
    Centre
St Mary's Hospital and University of
    Manchester
Manchester, UK

Justine Nugent MBBS MRCOG
Clinical Research Fellow
Maternal and Fetal Health Research
    Centre
St Mary's Hospital and University of
    Manchester
Manchester, UK

Lisa Penny MBChB MRCS Ed (A&E)
    FRCA
Specialist Registrar in Anaesthetics and
    Intensive Care
University Hospitals Birmingham
Queen Elizabeth Hospital
Birmingham, UK

Contributors

Rebekah Samangaya MBBS MRCOG
Specialist Registrar
Rochdale Hospital
Pennine Acute Hospitals NHS Trust
Rochdale, UK

Egidio da Silva MBChB, DA (UZ).
   FRCA (UK)
Specialist Registrar in Anaesthesia and
   Intensive Care
University Hospitals Birmingham
Queen Elizabeth Hospital
Birmingham, UK

Mark Tindall MBChB FRCA
Consultant in Anaesthesia
Dudley Group of Hospitals,
Dudley, West Midlands, UK

Clare Tower MBChB PhD MRCOG
Clinical Lecturer
Maternal and Fetal Health Research
   Centre
St Mary's Hospital and University of
   Manchester
Manchester, UK

Sarah Vause MD MRCOG
Consultant in Feto-Maternal Medicine
St Mary's Hospital
Manchester, UK

Foreword

Obstetric anaesthesia is a specialty interest within anaesthesia that has many features different from other areas of practice. Most obviously two patients, mother and baby, are affected by the same anaesthetic. Most of the mothers are healthy and are expecting a healthy baby as the end result of a straightforward physiological process. It is a very emotional time and is distressing when complications occur, especially if these are life-threatening to mother or baby. Most women remain awake through childbirth whether they have a vaginal or Caesarean delivery and often look to the anaesthetist for reassurance. The anaesthetist who is aware of the 'bigger picture' and knows about the complications that might occur and how the obstetrician and midwife will deal with them will be able to provide this reassurance with confidence.

The role of anaesthetists in obstetrics has changed over the years, such that it is now unthinkable that they were once regarded as mere technicians to deliver anaesthesia for an emergency Caesarean section and then leave the obstetric unit to fulfil duties elsewhere. Epidural analgesia during labour has become an expectation of many mothers and it is now used by almost one quarter of women. The obstetric anaesthetist is now an integral part of the maternity team where they need to be effective.

The importance of effective interdisciplinary working for maternity care is emphasised in all documents relating to standards and planning of maternity services. These include successive Confidential Enquiries into Maternal Deaths, *Safer Childbirth* and *Maternity Matters*. To be effective, the different disciplines need to understand the language and meaning that the other uses. This applies particularly to obstetrics, midwifery and anaesthesia but also to neonatal practice. As the title of this handbook implies it will be of immense value to the aspiring obstetric anaesthetist. I anticipate though that it will be equally useful to trainee obstetricians, midwives and paediatricians because the clarity of style and explanation of the implications of events mean that members of each discipline will understand the other.

Griselda Cooper OBE, FRCA, FRCOG

Preface

Anaesthetists on labour ward form an important part of a multi disciplinary team that includes obstetricians, midwives, paediatricians and theatre staff. This role is becoming ever important as anaesthetists now participate in the management of over 50% of patients in a typical unit. As well as traditional roles of providing analgesia and anaesthesia, anaesthetists are also involved in the acute management of conditions related to pregnancy, such as pre-eclampsia and major obstetric haemorrhage, and also coordinating and planning the care of patients with coexisting medical diseases.

Good communication on labour ward is vital to ensure clear, early decision making, and to be able to communicate the anaesthetist must be able to understand the basics of obstetrics. In common with most medical specialities obstetrics has terms and conditions unique to the speciality. In addition, there are a specialised set of procedures, many of which have important differences compared to normal medical and surgical practice. A lack of understanding of obstetric terminology and the significance of obstetricians' observations may lead to inefficient functioning of the team. Most anaesthetists, including trainees and consultants, have had no formal obstetric training since they were medical students.

The aim of this book is to provide anaesthetists with a basic knowledge of obstetrics and, more importantly, the implications this will have on their anaesthetic practice. This book is intended to complement, rather than replace, standard texts on obstetric anaesthesia and will hopefully provide a greater insight into the obstetric mysteries of labour ward!

We are keen to receive comments or suggestions about the book. Information regarding omissions or developments in practice are vital feedback. If you have useful information, or better approaches please contact us.

John Clift
Alexander Heazell

Acknowledgements

The editors would like to thank:

- All contributors for their hard work in preparation and execution of their manuscripts
- Mr Ben Jones for producing the photographic images within this handbook
- Mrs Betty Fulford at Cambridge University Press for her help, advice and support

Abbreviations

ACE	Angiotensin-converting enzyme
AFE	Amniotic fluid embolism
APH	Antepartum haemorrhage
APTT	Applied partial thromboplastin time
ARM	Artificial rupture of membranes
BMI	Body mass index
BP	Blood pressure
CEMACH	Confidential Enquiry into Maternal and Child Health
CNS	Central nervous system
CO	Cardiac output
CPR	Cardiopulmonary resuscitation
CS	Caesarean section
CSF	Cerebrospinal fluid
CT	Computerised tomography
CTG	Cardiotocograph
CVP	Central venous pressure
DIC	Disseminated intravascular coagulation
DVT	Deep vein thrombosis
ECG	Electrocardiograph
ECV	External cephalic version
EFM	Electronic fetal monitoring
FBC	Full blood count
FBS	Fetal blood sampling
FFP	Fresh frozen plasma
FHR	Fetal heart rate
FRC	Functional residual capacity
GBS	Group B streptococcus
HAART	Highly active antiretroviral therapy
Hb	Haemoglobin
HELLP	Haemolysis, elevated liver enzymes, low platelets
HDN	Haemolytic disease of the newborn
HIV	Human immunodeficiency virus
HSV	Herpes simplex virus
INR	International Normalized Ratio
IOL	Induction of labour
IUFD	Intrauterine fetal death
IUGR	Intrauterine growth restriction
IV	Intravenous
IM	Intramuscular

ITU	Intensive therapy unit
IVC	Inferior vena cava
LFT	Liver function tests
LOS	Lower oesophageal sphincter
LMWH	Low molecular weight heparin
LSCS	Lower segment Caesarean section
MAC	Minimum alveolar concentration
MAS	Meconium aspiration syndrome
NICE	National Institute for Health and Clinical Excellence
OP	Occipito-posterior
OT	Occipito-transverse
PE	Pulmonary embolism
PG	Prostaglandin
PPH	Postpartum haemorrhage
PROM	Pre-labour rupture of membranes
PT	Prothrombin time
PO	per oral
PR	per rectum
PV	per vagina
RBC	Red blood cells
RCOG	Royal College of Obstetricians and Gynaecologists
RCT	Randomised controlled trial
SC	Subcutaneous
SLE	Systemic lupus erythematosus
TED	Thromboembolic device
U & E	Urea and electrolytes
WCC	White cell count
VTE	Venous thromboembolism

Maternal physiology and obstetrics

John Clift

Overview of obstetrics

Obstetrics describes care related to pregnancy. In high-risk cases, such as maternal cardiac or renal disease, this may include pre-pregnancy care to optimise the mother's medical condition prior to conception. Care continues throughout the antenatal period, differing for women depending on their risk status (described in Chapter 2). Obstetric care then focuses on labour and delivery, and continues to the end of the postpartum period. During this time there are profound changes in maternal physiology. In addition, disorders may develop that are unique to pregnancy e.g. pre-eclampsia, obstetric cholestasis. An understanding of the changes in maternal physiology and the pathophysiology of pregnancy-related disorders is essential to provide safe, effective obstetric care.

Maternal physiology

There are many good textbooks describing the physiological changes occurring in pregnancy and these changes are beyond the scope of this book. This chapter summarises the implications these changes will have on anaesthetic practice.

Cardiovascular and haematological system

Changes to maternal cardiac physiology

- ↑ cardiac output (CO) (Figure 1.1), ↑ stroke volume, ↑ heart rate, ↓ systemic vascular resistance in pregnancy
- Left ventricular hypertrophy and dilatation
- Blood pressure alters throughout pregnancy (Figure 1.2)

    Patients with pre-existing cardiovascular disease decompensate during pregnancy and may develop cardiac failure. Auto-transfusion due to uterine emptying at delivery causes ↑ venous return, which may precipitate cardiac failure in susceptible patients.

- Patients with cardiovascular disease need close monitoring and multidisciplinary care throughout their pregnancy with the involvement of obstetricians, anaesthetists, intensivists and cardiologists

Obstetrics for Anaesthetists, ed. Alexander Heazell and John Clift. Published by Cambridge University Press. © Cambridge University Press 2008

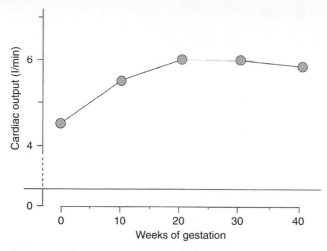

Figure 1.1 Cardiac output increases during the first trimester of pregnancy, remaining elevated throughout gestation. (Reproduced with permission from *ABC of Antenatal Care*, 4th edn, Blackwell Publishing, 2002.)[1]

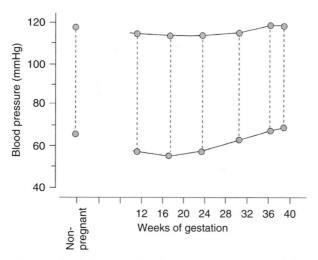

Figure 1.2 Blood pressure changes throughout pregnancy, falling during the first trimester, until approximately 20 weeks gestation, increasing towards or slightly above normal levels at 40 weeks gestation. (Reproduced with permission from *ABC of Antenatal Care*, 4th edn, Blackwell Publishing, 2002.)[1]

Uteroplacental circulation
- Receives 20% maternal CO at term
- Possesses no autoregulation properties
- Maternal hypotension, vasoconstriction and hypertonic uterine contractions decrease uteroplacental perfusion and may precipitate fetal hypoxia and distress

ECG
- Left axis deviation
- T waves may be inverted in lateral leads and lead III
- Mild tricuspid regurgitation may cause a grade I or II systolic murmur

Supine hypotensive syndrome
- Occurs from mid-pregnancy
- Gravid uterus compresses IVC, decreasing venous return and CO
- May cause placental hypoperfusion and maternal hypotension
- Avoid supine position, use left lateral position or left lateral tilt
- Worse with polyhydramnios and multiple pregnancies
- May be unmasked by regional or general anaesthesia

Blood pressure measurement in pregnancy
Mercury sphygmomanometry remains the most accurate method of measuring, although several automated machines have been validated to measure blood pressure in pregnancy.
- The optimal position is sitting although measuring the blood pressure in the left arm with the patient in the left lateral position is a useful alternative
- The diastolic blood pressure should be taken as the pressure at which the sounds disappear (the 5th Korotkov sound)
- A large cuff should be used if the patient's arm is greater than 33 cm in circumference

Circulating volume
- 45% ↑ plasma volume, 20% ↑ red cell mass, ↓ haemoglobin (Hb) from 13.3 to 10.9 g/dl = physiological anaemia of pregnancy (Figure 1.3)
- ↑ plasma volume delays the onset of signs and symptoms of hypovolaemia
- ↑ circulating volume allows compensation for average blood loss at vaginal delivery (300 ml) and Caesarean section (500 ml), negating the need for blood transfusion

Haematology
- ↑ WCC up to $10.5 \times 10^9/l$ in late pregnancy and as high as $20 \times 10^9/l$ in labour
- There is a slight ↓ platelet count during pregnancy

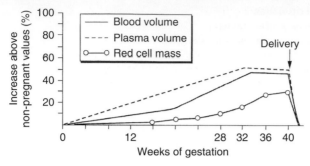

Figure 1.3 Increases in volume of constituents of blood during pregnancy, indicating that the largest component is expansion of plasma volume. (Reproduced with permission from *ABC of Antenatal Care*, 4th edn, Blackwell Publishing, 2002.)[1]

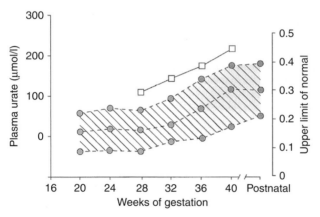

Figure 1.4 Concentration of urate in maternal plasma increases from the 20th week of gestation. There is a wide range of normal levels. ⊙ indicates the 10th, 50th and 90th centile values respectively; □ indicates elevated levels present in severe pre-eclampsia. (Reproduced with permission from *ABC of Antenatal Care*, 4th edn, Blackwell Publishing, 2002.)[1]

Clotting

- Patients are hypercoagulable to facilitate clotting at the time of placental separation and prevent bleeding during pregnancy
- ↑ all factors except XI and XIII
- Thromboembolic disease is leading cause of maternal mortality in the UK

- Consider thromboprophylaxis and/or early mobilisation in all patients
- ↑ risk of sagittal vein thrombosis

Biochemistry
- ↓ plasma urea and creatinine levels due to ↑ renal excretion
- Plasma urate 0.15–0.35 mmol/l (gestation dependent – see Figure 1.4)
- Liver enzymes are slightly elevated with a larger ↑ alkaline phosphatase secreted from placenta
- ↓ Ca^{2+}

Respiratory system

Oxygenation
- Functional residual capacity (FRC) ↓ by 20%, ↑ O_2 consumption by 20% at term (60% in labour) (Figure 1.5)
- Women desaturate much quicker when apnoeic (during attempts at intubation or eclamptic seizure)
- A pre-oxygenation period of 3–5 minutes is recommended before general anaesthetic

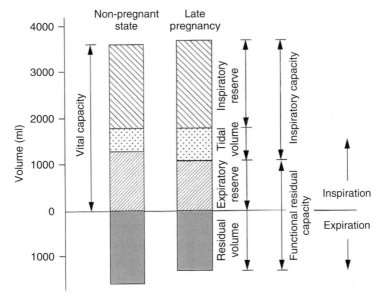

Figure 1.5 Changes in ventilatory volumes during pregnancy. (Reproduced with permission from *ABC of Antenatal Care*, 4th edn, Blackwell Publishing, 2002.)[1]

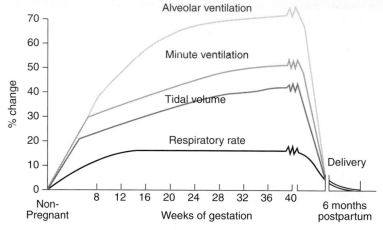

Figure 1.6 Changes in respiratory physiology during pregnancy, showing increased respiratory rate throughout pregnancy, and increasing tidal volume, minute and alveolar ventilation throughout pregnancy. (Reproduced from Buchan and Sharwood-Smith (1999)[2] with permission from *The Surgeon – Journal of the Royal Colleges of Surgeons of Edinburgh and Ireland*)

Ventilation

- ↑ tidal volume (TV), ↑ respiratory rate due to raised progesterone levels (Figure 1.6)
- ↓ $PaCO_2$ to 4.1 kPa; this needs maintaining during general anaesthesia, by increasing the minute volume by approximately 40%, to prevent maternal respiratory acidosis
- To compensate ↓ HCO_3^- (18–21 mmol/l) and base deficit −2 to −3

Hyperventilation

- During labour, minute ventilation may rise by up to 300%
- Left shift in O_2-dissociation curve causes ↑ maternal affinity for O_2 and a ↓ fetal O_2 delivery
- ↓ $PaCO_2$ may cause vasoconstriction between contractions resulting in a ↓ placental perfusion
- The above may be helped by epidural analgesia

Intubation in pregnancy

- Internal diameter of trachea decreased due to capillary engorgement of mucosa, therefore use a smaller endotracheal tube for a similar size non-pregnant woman
- Failed intubations 7–8 times more common in pregnancy, due to capillary engorgement and oedema of upper airway, increased chest diameter, large breasts,

increase in fat deposition, cricoid pressure, left lateral tilt and stress due to time demands

- Nasotracheal intubation and the insertion of nasopharyngeal airways should be avoided due to the increased risk of bleeding

Gastrointestinal system

- Progesterone-mediated ↓ LOS pressure and ↑ intra-abdominal pressure due to gravid uterus cause ↑ risk of reflux and aspiration of gastric contents
- Gastric emptying normal in pregnancy but delayed in labour and after administration of opiates
- Pregnant patients should be considered to be at risk from aspiration from approximately 16/40 (before if symptoms of reflux)
- Risk of regurgitation reduces to non-pregnant levels within 24–48 hours of delivery, provided there are no symptoms of reflux

Implications of changes in gastrointestinal physiology

- Patients should be premedicated with an H_2-blocking drug the evening before and on the morning of Caesarean section. 30ml 0.3 Mol sodium citrate should be given immediately before a rapid sequence induction with cricoid pressure, which is used when administering general anaesthesia.
- Many units have a policy of clear fluids only orally whilst in labour.

Central nervous system

Regional anaesthesia/analgesia

- ↑ lumbar lordosis, makes the interspinous spaces smaller making regional anaesthesia more difficult.
- ↑ sensitivity of nerves makes onset of block quicker and last longer.
- Distension of epidural veins increases risk of vascular damage/injection.
- 30–50% ↓ in doses of local anaesthetics for same block, compared with non-pregnant patients. Amongst proposed reasons are: engorged epidural veins may reduce the size of epidural space and the volume of CSF, swollen veins block the escape of drugs through the vertebral foramina, and cephalad spread due to exaggerated lumbar lordosis.

General anaesthetics

- MAC value of volatile anaesthetic agents ↓ by 25–40%
- ↓ sleep dose of thiopentone by approximately 35%
- The above are due to sedative effects of higher levels of progesterone, ↑ CNS serotonin activity and activation of endorphin system

Terms and definitions used in obstetrics

The specialised nature of obstetrics is associated with terms not used in other fields of medicine, for example, those that are used to describe the number of pregnancies and deliveries. The following list describes terms in common usage in obstetrics:

Gravidity The number of times a woman has been pregnant, irrespective of outcome.

Primigravida A woman who is pregnant for the first time.

Elderly primigravida A woman who is pregnant for the first time and is over 35 years of age.

Parity The number of times a woman has given birth to a fetus of 24 or more weeks gestation, irrespective of outcome/survival/mode of delivery.

Nulliparous A woman who has not given birth to a fetus of 24 or more weeks gestation.

Grandmultiparous A woman who has delivered 4 or more infants of 24 weeks gestation.

Gravida x *Para* y^{+z}

x = total number of pregnancies *including* present pregnancy

y = parity

z = the number of times a woman has been pregnant and not reached 24 weeks gestation e.g. miscarriages, ectopics

y^{+z} excludes the present pregnancy

Example: A woman currently pregnant having had one ectopic, one stillbirth at 27 weeks and one live baby is G4 P2^{+1}.

Antepartum Period between conception and the onset of labour, also known as the prenatal and antenatal period.

Intrapartum Time between the onset of labour and delivery of the placenta; during labour.

Postpartum Six-week period after childbirth during which the mother returns, physiologically, to her non-pregnant state. Also known as the puerperium and postnatal period.

Estimated date of delivery The day on which the baby is 'due', this is 40 weeks gestation. In most units this is now determined by ultrasound scanning in the first trimester; previously it was calculated as 40 weeks from the first day of the woman's last menstrual period.

X^{+y}/40 Shorthand method of writing gestation. X = number of weeks, y = number of days. Forty weeks is regarded as term.

Term $37^{+0} - 41^{+6}$ weeks' gestation.

Preterm (Premature) $24^{+0} - 36^{+6}$ weeks gestation i.e. less than 37 completed weeks' gestation.

Lie Describes the longitudinal axis of the fetus. Longitudinal lie – axis parallel with maternal spine, Transverse lie – axis at 90° with maternal spine, Oblique lie – in between longitudinal and transverse lie.

Presentation Part of fetus entering mother's pelvis first. Cephalic presentation – head; breech presentation – fetal foot, legs or bottom presents. Other presentations include face, brow, shoulder and compound (hand + presenting part).

Position Describes the position of the presenting part of the fetus with respect to the maternal pelvis. Cephalic presentations are described by the occiput. Occipito-anterior = fetal occiput facing anterior (symphysis), occipito-posterior = fetal occiput facing maternal posterior (sacrum), occipito-transverse = fetal occiput facing maternal side.

Rupture of membranes The membranes of the amniotic sac break releasing amniotic fluid per vagina.

Pre-labour rupture of membranes (PROM) > 37/40 gestation, rupture of membranes prior to onset of labour or contractions.

Preterm pre-labour rupture of membranes (PPROM) < 37/40 gestation, rupture of membranes prior to onset of labour or contractions.

Prolonged rupture of membranes Rupture of membranes more than 24 hours prior to the onset of labour.

Spontaneous rupture of membranes (SROM) > 37/40 gestation, rupture of membranes with or after the onset of labour.

Artificial rupture of membranes (ARM) Intentional rupturing of amniotic membranes with sterile instrument or finger sweep to induce labour. Also known as amniotomy.

External cephalic version (ECV) Procedure to externally rotate a breech presentation to cephalic. The fetal breech is disimpacted and the fetal head manipulated until cephalic. There is a higher success rate after 37 weeks.

Oligohydramnios A reduction in the volume of amniotic fluid surrounding the fetus. This may be caused by rupture of membranes, intrauterine growth restriction and renal/urogenital anomalies in the fetus.

Polyhydramnios Excessive amniotic fluid surrounding the fetus. This may be caused by gastrointestinal or neurological problems in the fetus, or maternal diabetes.

Low-birthweight baby An infant with a birthweight less than 2500 g.

Intrauterine growth restriction (IUGR) An infant that does not attain its predicted growth potential or an infant with a birthweight below the 5th centile for gestational age/ethnicity/parity.

Miscarriage Spontaneous loss of a pregnancy before 24 weeks gestation.

Tocolysis The suppression of uterine contractions.

Neonatal period The first 28 days of life.

Clinical implications

The following obstetric complications are increased in frequency in:
Primigravida

- Pre-eclampsia

Chapter 1

Elderly primigravida and women > 35
- Miscarriage
- Down's syndrome and chromosomal anomalies
- IUGR
- Premature labour
- Gynaecological disorders e.g. fibroids
- Other diseases e.g. ischaemic heart disease

High parity
- Abnormal fetal presentation
- Obstetric haemorrhage
- Uterine rupture during labour
- Grandmultiparous women have a 6 times increase in mortality rate compared with primigravida women

REFERENCES

1. G. Chamberlain and M. Morgan, *ABC of Antenatal Care, 4th edn* (Oxford: Blackwell Publishing, 2002).
2. A. S. Buchan and G. H. Sharwood-Smith *The Simpson Handbook of Obstetric Anaesthesia* (Edinburgh: Albamedia on behalf of The Royal College of Surgeons of Edinburgh, 1999). www.homepages.ed.ac.uk/asb/.

FURTHER READING

A. S. Buchan and G. H. Sharwood-Smith, *The Simpson Handbook of Obstetric Anaesthesia* (Edinburgh: Albamedia on behalf of The Royal College of Surgeons of Edinburgh, 1999). www.homepages.ed.ac.uk/asb/.

D. H. Chestnut, *Obstetric Anaesthesia Principles and Practice*, 3rd edn (New York: Mosby, 2004).

B. H. Heidemann and J. H. McClure, Changes in maternal physiology during pregnancy. *Continuing Education in Anaesthesia, Critical Care and Pain*, **3** (2003) 65–8.

I. Power and P. Kam, Maternal and Neonatal Physiology. In I. Power and P. Kam eds., *Principles of Physiology for the Anaesthetist* (London: Arnold Publishers, 2001).

Antenatal care

Clare Tower

The need for antenatal care

In 2003, the National Institute for Health and Clinical Excellence (NICE) produced guidelines for antenatal care provision, stating that modern antenatal care should fulfil the following functions:

- Identify risk factors
- Screening
- Education and modification of lifestyle
- Provide treatment and advice for minor ailments of pregnancy
- Psychological support and reassurance

Classification of high-risk and low-risk pregnancies

- The first antenatal visit or 'booking visit' is essential to identifying potential risk factors. Plans should be made and documented.
- Depending on the criteria used 19–50% of women will be defined as 'low' risk at booking.[1]
- This screening process should be ongoing and risk reassessed at each visit. This is particularly true of primiparous women.
- Most women in the UK attend for booking in the late first trimester or early second trimester. Those attending in the third trimester are likely to have risk factors placing them in a higher risk category.

The booking visit includes:

- Detailed history taking
- Appropriate clinical examination
- Maternal height and weight
- Blood pressure and urine examination
- Counselling and screening for infections, haematological disorders and fetal abnormalities
- Ultrasound scanning for dating and viability

High-risk patients with significant pre-existing diseases should be referred to an obstetric anaesthetist. Ideally at the first antenatal visit.

History

This should include:

- Previous pregnancies
- Maternal disease
- Family history

Obstetrics for Anaesthetists, ed. Alexander Heazell and John Clift. Published by Cambridge University Press. © Cambridge University Press 2008

Standardised checklists in maternity records aid this process, but the history should be taken by someone competent to identify risks and act accordingly. Despite this, studies have shown that risk factors present at booking are missed in up to 23% of pregnancies.[1]

Clinical examination

- Abdominal palpation and pelvic examination is generally unhelpful
- Cervical smear if indicated
- Examination of women who have previously undergone surgery or female genital mutilation
- Routine auscultation of maternal heart sounds is rarely of benefit in asymptomatic women
- Only women with a cardiac history, those with significant symptoms or immigrants require a full cardiovascular examination[1]
- Formal breast examination is not required[1]

Maternal height and weight

- Height and weight should be taken and body mass index (BMI) calculated (weight (kg)/height (m)^2). Maternal BMI is used for customised fetal growth charts that more accurately diagnose small-for-gestational-age babies.
- A BMI < 19 increases the risk of fetal growth restriction (FGR) and increases perinatal mortality.[2]
- Women of normal BMI do not require additional weight measurements.
- A BMI > 30 increases the risk of gestational diabetes, hypertension and large-for-dates infants with increased perinatal mortality.[3] Furthermore, analgesia during labour can be problematic due to technical difficulties with siting epidurals.

Assessment of blood pressure and urine

- Blood pressure (BP) should be measured at booking, then at each antenatal visit.
- In the first trimester BP $> 140/90$ mmHg on two occasions more than 2 hours apart should be investigated for an underlying renal, endocrine or collagen-vascular disorder.
- After 20 weeks gestation, screening is aimed at diagnosis of pre-eclampsia and gestational hypertension.
- Essential hypertension should only be diagnosed once these disorders have been excluded.
- Urine should be tested for protein, infection and glucose. Screening for asymptomatic bacteriuria reduces the risk of ascending infection.
- Glycosuria on more than one occasion warrants formal testing for gestational diabetes.

Screening for infection

- Pregnant women are offered screening for rubella, syphilis, hepatitis B and HIV.
- Rubella screening identifies women who require postnatal vaccination.
- Treatment of syphilis, hepatitis B and HIV improves fetal outcomes (see Chapter 11 on Infection).

Screening for fetal abnormalities

Screening policies for fetal abnormality vary from region to region. However, screening aims to identify:

- Anomalies that are incompatible with life
- Anomalies associated with increased morbidity and disability
- Treatable fetal conditions
- Fetal conditions that require monitoring and treatment after delivery

A detailed discussion of Down's syndrome screening is beyond the scope of this chapter. However, women are offered biochemical testing, ultrasound assessment of the nuchal translucency or both. The National Screening Committee suggested that women with a risk of 1:250 or more should be offered additional testing in the form of amniocentesis or chorionic villus sampling. Serum alpha-fetoprotein (AFP) testing in the second trimester is offered as a screening test for neural tube defects.

Ultrasound scanning

First trimester ultrasound aims to:

- Confirm a viable intra-uterine pregnancy
- Confirm gestation (as more accurate than last menstrual period), as this may reduce the need for induction of labour for post-maturity[4]
- Diagnose multiple pregnancy
- Diagnose and assess pelvic masses

Fetal ultrasound to identify structural abnormality is offered at 18–20 weeks' gestation.

Screening for haematological disorders

The following haematological disorders should be screened for:

- Anaemia

  The commonest cause of anaemia in pregnancy is iron deficiency, which should be treated. Further screening should be conducted at 28 and 34–36 weeks gestation. Normal haemoglobin levels are 11 g/dl in the first trimester falling to 10.5 g/dl at 28–32 weeks.

- Haemoglobinopathies (e.g. sickle cell anaemia/thalassaemia)

  This is now offered to all women regardless of ethnic group.

- Blood group and red cell alloantibodies
  All women (including rhesus-positive) should be screened for antibodies at booking, 28 and 34 weeks, as they may possess one of the non-rhesus red cell antibodies. Many units offer rhesus-negative women prophylactic anti-D at 28 and 34 weeks.

Antenatal care for the uncomplicated pregnancy

Hospital appointments

- The number and nature (midwife/GP/obstetrician) of antenatal appointments offered is not evidence based.
- Most women in the UK are offered 'shared care' between the community midwife, GP and hospital consultant.
- Obstetrician-based care is not associated with improved pregnancy outcome; thus in some regions low-risk women will be offered midwifery-led care, with referral to an obstetrician only if problems subsequently develop.
- A typical pattern of visits could be booking, 16 weeks, 20 weeks, monthly until 36 weeks, then weekly until delivery. At each visit BP, urine, symphysial fundal height for fetal growth, fetal presentation (third trimester only) and fetal heart auscultation are checked.

Ultrasonography

- Beyond scans at booking and for fetal anomaly, there is no indication for further scanning in an uncomplicated pregnancy.
- Ultrasound scanning is a useful tool in investigating problems suggested by clinical assessment, including diagnosis and monitoring of fetal growth and checking fetal presentation.

Antenatal care for complicated pregnancies

Multiple pregnancies

- Multiple pregnancies pose increased risk, thus require increased antenatal surveillance; most hospitals operate a specialist 'twin clinic'.
- Twins are classified as follows:

  > Dichorionic diamniotic (DCDA) – 2 separate pregnancies
  > Monochorionic diamniotic (MCDA) – 1 placenta, 2 amniotic sacs
  > Monochorionic monoamniotic (MCMA) – 1 placenta, 1 amniotic sac

- Determination of chorionicity is crucial to the planning of antenatal care. This can be reliably determined at 10–14 weeks gestation by ultrasound. Fifteen per cent of monochorionic twins develop twin–twin transfusion syndrome (TTTS) and hence are scanned regularly in the second trimester to enable early detection.[5]

- All twin pregnancies are at increased risk of IUGR, pre-eclampsia and anaemia, warranting more frequent antenatal checks of BP, urine and ultrasound scanning for fetal growth.

Pre-existing maternal medical conditions

Successful management of women with pre-existing medical disease requires a multidisciplinary approach, commonly in specialist clinics. This includes obstetricians, midwives, anaesthetists, intensivists, and consultants in the speciality relevant to the disease.

- Pre-pregnancy counselling is required to discuss maternal and fetal risk and to optimise drug treatment.
- An individualised package of antenatal care should be planned and documented at booking. There should be a method in place to ensure that all clinicians are informed of the treatment plan. Detailed discussion of individual cases is beyond the scope of this chapter, but key features of antenatal care are listed below.

There should be a method in place to ensure that all clinicians are informed of the treatment plan, and that it can be easily identified in the patient's notes by *all* those involved in patient care.

Cardiovascular disease

- Symptoms of cardiac disease are also those of normal pregnancy. For example, 75% of women complain of dyspnoea by 31 weeks, and women increase their heart rate by 20%.
- Benign ejection systolic murmurs may occur in up to 96% of pregnant women. The murmur is grade 1–2/6, midsystolic and heard loudest over the left sternal edge or pulmonary area. Other murmurs require investigation.
- Chest X-ray is safe with fetal shielding and should be performed if indicated.
- Echocardiography is safe and commonly performed to investigate cardiac function. Small pericardial effusions may be seen in 44% of normal pregnancies.
- Ideally, patients should be seen for pre-conceptual counselling so that teratogenic or fetotoxic drugs can be changed e.g. warfarin or ACE inhibitors.
- Screen for factors that contribute to cardiovascular decompensation, such as anaemia, infection and hypertension.

Specific cardiac conditions include:

Mitral stenosis

- Commonly due to rheumatic heart disease and should be considered in immigrants.
- Has 10–20 year asymptomatic phase so it may present for the first time in pregnancy with tachycardia and breathlessness.

- In severe cases, the maternal mortality is 5%.[6]
- The main complications are pulmonary oedema (especially immediately post-partum) and atrial fibrillation. Treatment is with diuretics and digoxin/beta-blockers respectively.
- Percutaneous balloon valvotomy is safe in pregnancy.
- Anticoagulation is required.

Congenital heart disease
- Increasing numbers of women who had surgery in childhood are now reaching reproductive age.
- Women with uncomplicated right-to-left shunts do well.
- Women with pulmonary hypertension, cyanosis and left ventricular outflow tract obstruction have a greater risk of problems.
- Pregnancy-induced fall in peripheral resistance increases right-to-left shunting and worsens cyanosis.
- Eisenmenger's syndrome is associated with a maternal mortality of 40%, thus women are advised against pregnancy and offered termination.
- Most maternal deaths occur during delivery and up to 1 week postpartum and are due to thromboembolism, pre-eclampsia or hypovolaemia.
- Thromboprophylaxis is required.
- Fetal echocardiography is required as there is an increased risk of fetal cardiac abnormality.
- Serial fetal growth scans in women with severe cardiac disease as there is increased risk of IUGR.
- Plans for mode and timing of delivery and anaesthesia are paramount.

Thrombophilia
- Can be inherited or acquired.
- Increased risks of thrombosis, pre-eclampsia, poor fetal growth, fetal loss and abruption.
- Risk depends on previous medical and obstetric history, family history and type of thrombophilia.
- A plan of care, including increased fetal surveillance, antenatal, intrapartum and postpartum thromboprophylaxis should be made early in pregnancy and involves the input of a haematologist. This should be clearly documented in the notes.
- To reduce the risks of epidural haematoma, regional techniques should not be used for 12 hours following a prophylactic dose of low molecular weight heparin (LMWH) or 24 hours after a therapeutic dose.
- LMWH should not be given for 4 hours after an epidural catheter has been inserted or removed and the catheter should not be removed within 10–12 hours of injection.

- Women on therapeutic doses should withhold the dose *the day before* elective Caesarean section or induction of labour e.g. 24 hrs between last dose and regional anaesthesia.
- Women on prophylactic doses should withhold the dose *on the day* of elective Caesarean section or induction of labour e.g. 12 hrs between last dose and regional anaesthesia.
- Women should be advised to stop injections as soon as she thinks she may be in labour and arrange early medical contact.

> Discussions should take place between the haematologists, obstetricians and anaesthetists coordinating the administration of heparin to facilitate the timing of delivery to allow the use of regional anaesthesia and elective surgery.

Renal disease

- Risks depend on the degree of renal impairment and complications such as hypertension, proteinuria and infection.
- Management is individualised and involves renal physicians.
- Pre-pregnancy serum creatinine is used to aid management. Women with a serum creatinine $< 120\,\mu mol/l$ have a small risk of long-term renal damage as a result of pregnancy, whereas those with severely impaired renal function (creatinine $> 175\,\mu mol/l$) have much greater risks of permanent deterioration.
- Close monitoring of proteinuria, BP, renal function and testing for urinary infection.
- Serial fetal growth scans are needed as risks of pre-eclampsia and IUGR are increased.
- Women on dialysis are at risk of preterm delivery.
- Discussion of drug therapy in women with renal transplants is needed. Prednisolone, azathioprine and cyclosporin have all been taken throughout pregnancy without significant increased fetal risk, although cyclosporin may be associated with IUGR.

Diabetes mellitus (DM)

- Should be managed in a specialist clinic involving specialist nurses and diabetologists.
- Increased risk of fetal abnormality is related to degree of glycaemic control at conception.
- Increased risk of abnormal fetal growth (usually macrosomia), thus third trimester serial scans are required.
- Increased risks of pre-eclampsia.
- Maternal insulin requirements commonly increase during pregnancy.
- Good diabetic control improves obstetric outcome.

Respiratory disorders
- Asthma is the commonest respiratory disorder encountered in pregnancy.
- Outcome is better in women with good asthma control preconception.
- Deterioration is commoner in the third trimester due to effects of the growing fetus.
- Reassurance that medication should continue and does not pose a risk to the fetus is paramount.

Pregnancy-related maternal conditions

Hypertension
- Defined as BP $> 140/90$ mmHg on two occasions 4 hours apart.
- Pre-eclampsia is defined as hypertension after 20 weeks associated with proteinuria > 300 mg/24 hours that resolves postpartum.
- Gestational hypertension or pregnancy-induced hypertension is hypertension after 20 weeks but without proteinuria.
- All women with raised BP warrant additional monitoring due to the increased risks of pre-eclampsia.
- At present there is no universal antenatal screening test able to predict the development of pre-eclampsia. Some units utilise uterine artery Doppler in high-risk women.
- Proteinuria may develop before hypertension; thus persistent isolated protein-uria warrants further investigation.
- Investigations include ultrasound assessment of the fetus, liver and renal func-tion tests (including urate), full blood count (FBC) and clotting. A 24-hour urinary collection for protein is required for certain diagnosis, along with a midstream specimen of urine to exclude urinary tract infection.
- Some women may require treatment with antihypertensives such as labetalol, nifedipine or methyldopa.

Obstetric cholestasis
- Obstetric cholestasis is a poorly understood disease of pregnancy associated with maternal pruritus, raised bile acids and abnormal liver enzymes.
- Monitoring of bile acids, liver enzymes and regular fetal assessment is required.
- Ursodeoxycholic acid may relieve maternal itching and improve liver function results.
- Vitamin K supplementation after 36 weeks is needed.
- It is associated with late intrauterine fetal death (IUFD) (after 38 weeks), thus delivery at 37–38 weeks is offered.

A clotting profile is needed in patients with cholestasis prior to regional anaes-thesia/analgesia.

Thrombocytopenia

- Occurs in 5–10% of women at term, 75% of which have gestational/pregnancy-associated thrombocytopenia.
- Gestational thrombocytopenia is benign and there are no adverse outcomes even if platelets fall to $<100 \times 10^9/l$. No intervention is required.
- Other more serious causes should be excluded.
- Thrombocytopenia present in the first half of pregnancy is more likely to be due to chronic immune thrombocytopenia (ITP).
- Haemorrhage is unlikely with platelet counts $>50 \times 10^9/l$, and spontaneous haemorrhage unlikely with counts $>20 \times 10^9/l$.
- Platelet counts are monitored 2–4 weekly.
- Fetus is at risk (albeit low) of thrombocytopenia and associated bleeding. This is unrelated to the maternal platelet count, so at risk fetuses cannot be identified antenatally.
- Caesarean section is carried out only for obstetric complications.
- Treatment is steroids or immunoglobulins.

Recommended thresholds are $> 50 \times 10^9/l$ for vaginal delivery and $> 80 \times 10^9/l$ for epidural and Caesarean section.

Gestational diabetes mellitus

- Associated with adverse obstetric outcome as previously discussed.
- Usual stepwise management of diet, oral hypoglycaemics and insulin is followed.

Anaemia

- Anaemia should be treated with iron and folate supplementation.
- Risks of blood loss at delivery should be remembered.
- Women with thalassaemia traits require folate supplementation.
- The maximum rise in haemoglobin with oral supplementation is 0.8 g/dl per week.
- Severe anaemia may need parenteral iron or blood transfusion prior to delivery.

The role of the anaesthetist in the antenatal clinic/day assessment unit

In many obstetric units, anaesthetists run a specialist clinic for the review of antenatal patients. This care is geared towards anticipating problems at delivery and planning accordingly in order to minimise risk.

Cases recommended for referral to an anaesthetist:
- Previous anaesthetic problems (general, spinal or epidural)
- Neurological disorders
- Severe respiratory disorders
- All cardiovascular/cardiac disorders
- Renal disorders
- Liver disorders
- Rheumatological disease
- Haematological disease
- Anticoagulated patients
- Jehovah's witnesses
- Porphyria
- Morbid obesity
- Patients with back problems e.g. trauma/previous surgery
- Patients with obstetric problems increasing the risk of Caesarean section or haemorrhage e.g multiple pregnancies, pre-eclampsia etc.
- Patients wishing to discuss anaesthesia or analgesia
- Any patient who midwifery staff or obstetricians think should be reviewed by an anaesthetist

REFERENCES

1. K. Chan and L. Kean, Routine antenatal care at the booking clinic. *Curr. Obstet. Gynaecol.*, **14**:2 (2004), 79–85.
2. D.A. Doherty, E.F. Magann, J. Francis, J.C. Morrison and J.P. Newnham, Pre-pregnancy body mass index and pregnancy outcomes. *Int. J. Gynaecol. Obstet.*, **95**:3 (2006), 247–7.
3. R. Fraser and K. Chan, Problems of obesity in obstetric care. *Curr. Obstet. Gynaecol.*, **13**:4 (2003), 239–43.
4. J. Gardosi, T. Vanner and A. Francis, Gestational age and induction of labour for prolonged pregnancy. *Br. J. Obstet. Gynaecol.*, **104**:7 (1997), 792–7.
5. P. Vankayalapati and B. Hollis, Role of ultrasound in obstetrics. *Curr. Obstet. Gynaecol.*, **14** (2004), 92–8.
6. J.Y.-L. Tan, Cardiovascular disease in pregnancy. *Curr. Obstet. Gynaecol.*, **14** (2004), 155–65.

FURTHER READING

Antenatal screening for Down's Syndrome – Policy and Quality Issues. June 2003. National Screening Committee. www.screening.nhs.uk

National Institute for Health and Clinical Excellence, *Antenatal care: routine care for the healthy pregnant women.* Clinical Guideline (London: Department of Health, 2003). www.nice.org.uk.

Nelson-Piercy, Handbook of Obstetric Medicine, 3rd edn. (London: Taylor and Francis, 2006).

Royal College of Obstetricians and Gynaecologists, *Thromboprophylaxis During Pregnancy, Labour and After Vaginal Delivery*. Guideline Number 37. (London: RCOG Press, 2004).

Induction of labour

Rebekah Samangaya

Introduction

Induction of labour is defined as an intervention to artificially initiate uterine contractions to lead to cervical effacement and dilatation, and delivery of the baby. This definition incorporates women with intact membranes and those with spontaneous rupture of membranes who have not gone into labour. In the UK, about 20% of pregnancies are induced.

Indications for induction of labour

The indications for induction of labour (IOL) can be divided into fetal or maternal indications. It is important that IOL is initiated for a specific indication, due to the associated risks. The benefits of delivery should outweigh the risks of continuing the pregnancy.

Fetal

Post maturity

Prolonged pregnancy is the most common indication for IOL. Guidelines from the National Institute for Health and Clinical Excellence (NICE)[1] recommend offering IOL to women between 41 and 42 weeks' gestation. This gestation is utilised due to the risk of stillbirth rising from 1 per 1000 pregnancies at 42 weeks to 2 per 1000 pregnancies at 43 weeks. Prolonged gestation can also be associated with an increase in intrapartum complications such as fetal distress.

Suspected fetal compromise

Suspected fetal compromise may be an indication for IOL. Placental insufficiency including intrauterine growth restriction (IUGR), reduced liquor volume, or an abnormal Doppler ultrasound of the umbilical artery is an indication for delivery of the baby, as is rhesus incompatibility where the fetus may be at risk of anaemia.

Women with a history of recurrent antepartum haemorrhages (APH) may be induced around term, as such a history may be suggestive of recurrent small placental abruptions and may predispose to placental insufficiency.

Neonatal care

Some babies will require specialist neonatal services, such as surgery in the early neonatal period. In such cases women should be induced at a suitable unit with specialist staff and facilities, at an appropriate time of day.

Obstetrics for Anaesthetists, ed. Alexander Heazell and John Clift. Published by Cambridge University Press © Cambridge University Press 2008

Controversial indications

Suspected fetal macrosomia has in the past been an indication for IOL. However, ultrasound scans will have a variance of $+/-15\%$ when estimating fetal weight. Randomised trials comparing expectant management to IOL in suspected fetal macrosomia in non-diabetic women have demonstrated no benefit in terms of instrumental delivery or Caesarean section rates and no change in perinatal mortality.[2]

Maternal

Medical conditions

Maternal diabetes is associated with a rise in perinatal mortality rate and stillbirth. In addition these women are more likely to have a baby that is macrosomic with possible implications for a difficult delivery. Therefore, women with pre-existing diabetes are often induced at or beyond 38 weeks gestation. There is more uncertainty regarding induction of labour before 38 weeks gestation in women with gestational diabetes.

For women with pre-eclampsia, the ultimate treatment is delivery. Therefore, these women will often be induced. The timing of this will depend on the gestation at which pre-eclampsia has developed as well as the severity, and urgency of delivery. Women with a history of stillbirth are often offered IOL before term, in an attempt to alleviate anxiety.

Pre-labour rupture of membranes

Pre-labour rupture of membranes (PROM) occurs in about 10% of term pregnancies. Most women (86%) with ruptured membranes at term will progress into spontaneous labour within 24 hours. The main risk for women with prolonged ruptured membranes is intra-uterine infection. Although expectant management may be utilised for the first 24–48 hours, it is recommended that women are delivered within 96 hours of membrane rupture.

Women with PROM are more likely to have:
- Chorioamnionitis
- Retained placenta
- Primary or secondary postpartum haemorrhage

Maternal request

Maternal request may be a valid indication for IOL, provided there is a clear underlying reason. However, it is important to fully counsel such women on the potential risks of IOL including increased rate of Caesarean and instrumental vaginal delivery.

Table 3.1 Examples of high-risk cases for induction of labour

Fetal	Maternal
Suspected IUGR	Previous Caesarean section
Fetal abnormality requiring neonatal specialist care e.g. gastroschisis	Pre-eclampsia
	High parity
Suspected fetal infection	Diabetes mellitus
Twins	

Timing and location of induction of labour

Maternity units throughout the UK have different policies on timing of IOL and the location where induction is commenced. There may be some benefit in commencing IOL in the morning as opposed to the evening.[3] Some maternity units conduct all inductions on the delivery suite, although the majority of units will administer prostaglandins in low-risk cases on the antenatal wards. In high-risk cases IOL is usually performed on delivery suites (Table 3.1).

Patient assessment

Prior to commencing IOL, the obstetric history should be reviewed to confirm there are no contraindications. It is important to determine that the woman is fully aware of the process, the potential risks and the possible duration. An abdominal examination is performed to confirm that the fetus is in a cephalic presentation, and that the head is at least partially engaged into the pelvis. A vaginal examination should be performed to assess the cervical ripeness, since the method of induction is dependent on the cervical ripeness on vaginal examination. A lower score is associated with increased risk of Caesarean section. Cervical ripeness is often assessed using the modified Bishop's score (Table 3.2).

A lower Bishop's score is associated with increased risk of Caesarean section

Methods of induction of labour

Membrane sweep

Women are offered a membrane sweep at or beyond term, which is an intervention that can be easily done in hospital or community-based clinics. This involves a vaginal examination where a finger is inserted through the cervix, and the membranes swept off the uterine wall around the cervix. Sweeping of the membranes is associated with a reduced duration of pregnancy, and requirement for formal

Table 3.2 Modified Bishops' score

	Score		
	0	1	2
Station of head in relation to ischial spines	-3	-2	$-1,0$
Cervical dilatation (cm)	Closed	1–2	3–4
Length of cervix (cm)	>2	1–2	<1
Cervical consistency	Firm	Medium	Soft
Position of cervix	Posterior	Mid-position	Anterior

Table 3.3 Formulations of PGE_2 for use in induction of labour

Formulation	Dose	Frequency	Maximum dose
PGE_2 tablets	3 mg	6–8hourly	6 mg
PGE_2 gels	2 mg – nulliparous women with unfavourable cervix	6hourly	4 mg – nulliparous women with unfavourable cervix
	1 mg – all other women		3 mg – other women

induction.[4,5] Membrane sweep should be avoided if there is evidence of a low-lying placenta or a history of significant APH.

Prostaglandins

Prostaglandins are utilised to ripen the cervix, and are given in preference to oxytocin to nulliparous or multiparous women with intact membranes. In women with PROM, prostaglandins or oxytocin can be given dependent on Bishop's score. Vaginal prostaglandins can be given as either tablet or gel formulations. The regimes for these two preparations are demonstrated in Table 3.3.[1]

Vaginal prostaglandins can be safely given on antenatal wards, provided the fetus is monitored by electronic fetal monitoring for approximately 30 minutes prior to administration of the prostaglandin and 1 hour after. High-risk cases, for example where there is evidence of fetal compromise, are often undertaken on delivery suites.

Recent trials have explored the use of misoprostol (PGE_1). Misoprostol can be kept at room temperature, unlike PGE_2 preparations, which are refrigerated, and thus may be a more useful preparation in poorer areas of the world. In addition, misoprostol can be given orally as well as vaginally, which is often preferred by women. Misoprostol appears to be as effective as PGE_2 preparations in both vaginal and oral forms,[6,7] although there are concerns about an increase in uterine hyperstimulation.[7,8] At present, misoprostol is not used routinely in the UK for IOL.

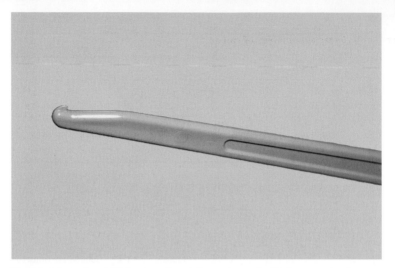

Figure 3.1 Device for artificial rupture of amniotic membranes (ARM), the external surfaces are smooth to prevent damage to maternal or fetal tissues.

Artificial rupture of membranes/amniotomy

Following cervical ripening with prostaglandins, artificial rupture of membranes (ARM) is performed to initiate labour. An ARM is usually performed on the delivery suite, using a sterile device with a sharp edge shielded from the baby (see Figure 3.1). On occasions ARM may be done in theatre. The main indication for an ARM in theatre is a high presenting fetal head, and therefore a significant risk of cord prolapse. Some women with prolonged ruptured membranes may still have forewaters intact and still require an ARM. After an ARM, women may proceed into labour, but many will require an oxytocin infusion. The time interval between amniotomy and commencing oxytocin will depend on individual preferences. Parous women are more likely to begin contracting after an ARM than primigravidae, and therefore a regime often followed is to commence oxytocin 1 hour after amniotomy in primigravidae and 2 hours after in multiparous women.

> ARM should be done in theatre if high presenting fetal head because of an increased risk of cord prolapse. Anaesthetist should be informed and prepared to anaesthetise for category 1 Caesarean section if cord prolapse does occur.

Oxytocin

Before commencing oxytocin, it is important to ensure that the membranes are ruptured. Oxytocin may be used alone, or following vaginal prostaglandins.

The regimes used for oxytocin administration vary in different maternity units, although recently NICE guidelines have recommended a standardised dilution should be implemented. Oxytocin is commenced at 1 mUnit/ min, and increased at time intervals of 30 minutes. The rate of oxytocin is titrated according to the frequency of contractions, aiming for about 3–4 contractions in 10 minutes. Women on oxytocin infusions should have continuous electronic fetal monitoring.

Women who are undergoing IOL may request an epidural prior to artificial rupture of membranes or commencement of oxytocin.

Complications of induction of labour

Failed induction of labour

In some women, prostaglandins have no effect, such that there is no improvement on the cervical ripeness. If the cervix is unfavourable to the extent that the membranes cannot be ruptured, the reason for IOL should be reassessed. For some women waiting a few more days may help, but in others the only viable option is to consider a Caesarean section.

Analgesia requirements

There is an increase in requirement for pain relief in women that are being induced, and analgesia will be requested earlier in labour as compared to spontaneous labours. This is partly related to the longer time period that women may be in pain, but also to the nature of the pain.

Epidural analgesia is associated with a longer labour in women that are induced.[9]

There is an increase in the rate of epidural analgesia in women who have IOL.[10]

Fetal distress

Induction of labour is associated with an increased incidence of non-reassuring fetal heart patterns,[9] and therefore all women undergoing IOL should have continuous external fetal monitoring during labour, and whilst on oxytocin.

Uterine hyperstimulation (see Chapter 5 on Abnormal labour)

Uterine hyperstimulation can occur with PGE_2, PGE_1 or oxytocin, and can result in fetal distress or a fetal bradycardia in the case of a prolonged contraction. The infusion rate of oxytocin is titrated according to the frequency and strength of contractions, and so should be reduced if there is hyperstimulation. If there is a sustained contraction, or hyperstimulation with PGE_2 or PGE_1, tocolytics such as sublingual glyceryl trinitrate, inhaled salbutamol or subcutaneous terbutaline can be used.

Instrumental delivery

Women that are induced have a higher risk of instrumental delivery.[11] This may be due to an increase in suspected fetal distress, but other confounding factors like the use of epidurals and prolonged labour may also have an effect.

Caesarean section

The requirement for Caesarean is increased in women that are induced.[10] This may be due to the increase in suspected fetal distress, or an increase in failure to progress.

> **Anaesthetic implications:**
> IOL increases risk of:
> * Caesarean section
> * Instrumental delivery
> * Fetal distress

High-risk cases

Previous Caesarean section

Women with a past history of Caesarean section are at increased risk of uterine rupture, and this risk is increased with IOL.[12] This risk is increased by using both prostaglandins and oxytocin. Uterine rupture or scar dehiscence is associated with significant maternal and perinatal morbidity and mortality (see Chapter 9).

High parity

Grand multiparous women (who have delivered 5 or more babies) are at an increased risk of uterine rupture. Prostaglandin E_2 formulations or oxytocin can be associated with hyperstimulation, which increases the risk of uterine rupture.

Pre-eclampsia

Women with pre-eclampsia are more susceptible to fluid overload. Oxytocin is usually diluted in normal saline, and women can receive substantial volumes if they are on maximum rates for a long period of time. In addition, oxytocin as an antidiuretic will reduce urine output. To reduce the volume of fluid given, women with pre-eclampsia should receive double concentration intravenous oxytocin, at half the infusion rate.

Twins

Women with twins may be induced at around 38 weeks gestation due to maternal discomfort. In addition, there is an increase in risk of stillbirth in multiple pregnancies, and so such pregnancies are unlikely to go beyond term.

High presenting fetal part

As previously discussed, women with a high presenting fetal head may require an ARM in theatre due to the risk of cord prolapse. Women with an unstable lie may have the lie stabilised to a cephalic longitudinal presentation and an ARM performed in theatre. In all these cases, until the woman is contracting strongly, there will be a risk of cord prolapse, and such women will require continuous fetal monitoring.

Intra-uterine fetal death

Intrauterine fetal death (IUFD) may occur at any stage of pregnancy. The causes of IUFD include fetal anomalies, infection, fetal hypoxia secondary to placental insufficiency.[13] The cause of the majority of cases of IUFD is unknown. Intrauterine fetal death should be confirmed by two obstetricians or ultrasonographers, and is confirmed by visualisation of the inactive fetal heart.

Unless there is risk to maternal health, IUFD should be delivered vaginally. Indications for Caesarean section include maternal haemorrhage (e.g. massive placental abruption) or severe pre-eclampsia/eclampsia/HELLP syndrome. For vaginal delivery, women should be given mifepristone (an anti-progesterone, also known as RU486) 200 mg.[14] After 24–36 hours a prostaglandin, either gemeprost, PGE_1 or PGE_2 should be given. This regime may need to be supplemented with oxytocin.

Women with IUFD have to deal with a combination of grief and labour pain, so every effort should be made to support the woman and her partner at this time, and provide adequate analgesia.

- Epidural analgesia is often used for labour in patients with IUFD
- Platelets and clotting should be checked prior to administration of epidural as IUFD is associated with maternal coagulopathy[15]
- Incidence of coagulopathy increases with duration of period since fetal demise

REFERENCES

1. National Institute for Health and Clinical Excellence. *Inherited Clinical Guideline D. Induction of Labour.* (London: Department of Health, 2001).
2. O. Irion and M. Boulvain, Induction of labour for suspected fetal macrosomia. *Cochrane Database Syst. Rev.*, **2** (2000), CD000938.
3. J. M. Dodd, C. A. Crowther and J. S. Robinson, Morning compared with evening induction of labour: a nested randomized controlled trial. *Obstet. Gynecol.*, **108**:2 (2006), 350–60.
4. E. de Miranda, J. van der Bom, G. J. Bonsel, O. P. Bleker and F. R. Rosendaal, Membrane sweeping and prevention of post-term pregnancy in low-risk pregnancies: a randomised controlled trial. *BJOG*, **113** (2006), 402–8.

5. M. Boulvain, C. Stan and O. Irion, Membrane sweeping for induction of labour. *Cochrane Database Syst. Rev.*, **1** (2005), CD000451.

6. J. M. Dodd, C. A. Crowther and J. S. Robinson, Oral misoprostol for induction of labour at term: randomised controlled trial. *BMJ*, **332** (2006), 509–13.

7. G. J. Hofmeyr and A. M. Gulmezoglu, Vaginal misoprostol for cervical ripening and induction of labour. *Cochrane Database Syst. Rev.*, 1 (2003), CD000941.

8. Z. Alfirevic and A. Weeks, Oral misoprostol for induction of labour. *Cochrane Database Syst. Rev.*, **1** (2006), CD001338.

9. N. Rojansky, V. Tanos, B. Reubinoff, S. Shapira and D. Weinstein, Effect of epidural analgesia on duration and outcome of induced labour. *Int. J. Gynaecol. Obstet.*, **56** (1997), 237–44.

10. J. C. Glantz, Elective induction vs. spontaneous labor associations and outcomes. *J. Reprod. Med.*, **50**:4 (2005), 235–40.

11. C. Mazouni, G. Porcu, F. Bretelle *et al.*, Risk factors for forceps delivery in nulliparous patients. *Acta Obstet. Gynecol. Scand.*, **85** (2006), 298–301.

12. S. I. Kayani and Z. Alfirevic, Uterine rupture after induction of labour in women with previous caesarean section. *BJOG*, **112**:4 (2005), 451–5.

13. J. Gardosi, S. M. Kady, P. McGeown, A. Francis and A. Tonks, Classification of stillbirth by relevant condition at death (ReCoDe): population based cohort study. *BMJ*, **331** (2005), 1113–17.

14. R. Frydman, H. Fernandez, J. C. Pons *et al.*, Mifepristone (RU486) and therapeutic late pregnancy termination: a double blind study of two different doses. *Hum. Reprod.*, **3** (1988), 803–6.

15. A. D. Maslow, T. W. Breen, M. C. Sarna *et al.*, Prevalence of coagulation abnormalities associated with intrauterine fetal death. *Can. J. Anaesth.*, **43**:12 (1996), 1237–43.

Normal labour

Sarah Vause

Introduction

Labour is a physiological process and as such there are times when it may work efficiently and times when it may be dysfunctional. By monitoring the process of labour we aim to detect deviations from normality, and intervene appropriately. Whilst appropriate interventions, at the appropriate time, promote maternal and fetal wellbeing, inappropriate, unnecessary or badly timed interventions may compromise it.

Throughout this chapter a distinction will be drawn between nulliparous and multiparous women. Multiparous women have a more compliant cervix and faster progress in labour can be anticipated.

Definition of labour – stages of labour

There is no standard definition of labour. However most suggested definitions incorporate progressive effacement and dilatation of the cervix in the presence of regular painful uterine contractions.

Labour can be divided into three stages:
- First stage – Onset of labour until full dilatation of the cervix (10 cm)
- Second stage – Full dilatation of the cervix until delivery of the baby
- Third stage – Delivery of the baby until delivery of the placenta

First stage of labour
The first stage can be further divided into the latent phase (early labour) and active phase (established labour) (Figure 4.1).

During the latent phase the cervix is changing (softening and effacing) but often shows little change in dilatation. In primiparous women the cervix usually becomes completely effaced before dilating, whereas in multiparous women the cervix may begin to dilate before effacement is complete.

Second stage
The onset of second stage is diagnosed by finding the cervix fully dilated (10 cm). The vaginal examination may be performed because a fixed amount of time has elapsed since the previous vaginal examination, or because the woman has an urge to push or the fetal presenting part is visible.

The second stage can be divided into the passive and active phases. The passive phase lasts from diagnosis of full dilatation until the woman begins to push or the

Obstetrics for Anaesthetists, ed. Alexander Heazell and John Clift. Published by Cambridge University Press. © Cambridge University Press 2008

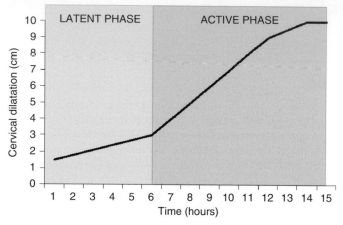

Figure 4.1 Graphical representation of cervical dilatation in the first stage of labour, showing progressive dilatation during the active phase of labour (darker background).

fetal presenting part is visible. The active second stage is the time when the woman is actively pushing. During the active second stage the woman is exerting herself by performing repeated Valsalva manoeuvres, maternal cardiac output is approximately 9–10 l/min and fetal pH falls progressively.

Distension of the pelvic floor by the fetal head initiates Ferguson's reflex which gives a woman the urge to push. When regional analgesia is used this reflex is often abolished.

Third stage

The third stage of labour lasts from delivery of the baby until expulsion of the placenta. Active management of the third stage of labour (oxytocin or Syntometrine, combined with early clamping of the umbilical cord and delivery of the placenta by controlled cord traction) reduces the risk of postpartum haemorrhage.

Onset and mechanism of labour

Onset of labour

In humans no single mechanism for the initiation of labour has been identified. There appears to be an interaction between the fetal pituitary–adrenal axis and the placenta. The changes in placental function in turn down-regulate the factors that keep the uterus quiescent during pregnancy and alter the maternal hormonal balance in favour of parturition. At term, the fetus increases its production of cortisol and this cortisol reduces the production of placental progesterone and increases the production of oestrone and oestradiol. Progesterone suppresses uterine activity and oestradiol increases it. Increased numbers of gap junctions form between the myocytes allowing intracellular communication and production of coordinated contractions. Pro-inflammatory cytokines are released which increase prostaglandin release. This leads to cervical ripening, a process mimicked by prostaglandin administration for induction of labour. Prostaglandins potentiate the action of oxytocin, which enhances myometrial activity.

Mechanism of labour

The fetal head usually enters the pelvis in a transverse position because the pelvic inlet is widest in the transverse diameter. During normal labour the fetal head flexes and rotates to an occipito-anterior (OA) position as it descends through the pelvis. The maternal pelvic outlet is widest in the antero-posterior diameter. This provides the best fit for the fetal head as it traverses the maternal pelvis. Obstruction to the process of labour can occur if a fetal head is deflexed, or fails to rotate in the usual way. This obstruction can be relative or absolute.

As the fetal head crowns on the perineum, extension of the head occurs. This is then followed by restitution of the fetal head to its normal position with respect to the fetal shoulders. The fetal shoulders deliver in the antero-posterior diameter, the anterior shoulder delivering first followed by the posterior shoulder. The rest of the body normally follows easily.

Following delivery of the baby, contraction of the uterus produces placental separation and expulsion. There is a concomitant auto-transfusion of approximately 500 ml of blood from the contracting uterus into the maternal circulation.

Duration of normal labour

First stage

The latent phase of labour may stop and start, and may take several hours or days. Women often regard themselves as being in labour and can find a long latent phase tiring and distressing. A long latent phase is more common in primiparous women than multiparas.[1]

The active phase or established labour commences at 3–4 cm dilatation, after which progress at a rate of 1 cm per hour is expected, these figures have been derived from work done by Friedman in the 1950s.[2,3,4] Although others have subsequently suggested other slightly different figures, 1 cm per hour remains the 'rule of thumb' in the majority of labour wards. Multiparous women tend to progress more quickly than primiparous women. Therefore, slow progress in a multiparous woman is more significant than in a primipara.

The diagnosis of the onset of labour is important.

Unnecessary intervention for slow progress may occur if the onset of labour is incorrectly diagnosed.

The frequency of vaginal examinations varies according to the policy of different hospitals, but is usually *at least every four hours*.

If a woman makes less than 2 cm progress between vaginal examinations 4 hours apart she would be deemed to be making slow progress.[5]

Second stage

There is little agreement about the normal duration of the second stage of labour, particularly the passive second stage. Duration is dependent on the presence of regional analgesia, policies relating to the frequency of vaginal examinations and hospital protocols relating to the commencement of directed pushing. There does not appear to be a significant risk from waiting up to two hours before the commencement of pushing, and it may allow time for the fetal head to descend and rotate. Trials have shown that this does not reduce the overall operative delivery rate but may reduce the need for rotational instrumental vaginal delivery.[6]

During the active second stage, most women are unable to push effectively for more than an hour. Progress in second stage is assessed by the descent and position of the fetal head. Women are usually examined, with a view to assessing whether operative delivery is indicated, after an hour of active pushing.

Regional analgesia leads to:

Relaxation of the pelvic floor muscles – leading to more occipito-posterior (OP) and occipito-transverse (OT) positions

Decreased sensation of Ferguson's reflex – loss of urge to push

When a patient has regional analgesia and is fully dilated an additional hour is allowed during the second stage of labour for passive descent and rotation of the fetal head.

Third stage

The third stage of labour is delayed, if not completed within half an hour of birth with active management.[5] Some women prefer a more natural or conservative approach to the management of the third stage. If this "physiological" management is chosen, this time limit of 30 minutes does not apply.

Interpreting a partogram

The partogram is a chart that summarises the maternal and fetal monitoring during labour (Figure 4.2). Maternal pulse, blood pressure, temperature, urine output and urinalysis are charted. Fetal heart rate and the colour of the liquor are charted. It usually also contains a record of intravenous fluids and drugs given.

The partogram differs from a normal observation chart in that it also includes a chart to plot the progress of labour including contraction frequency and strength, cervical dilatation and descent of the fetal head.

Research has shown that the use of a partogram helps to detect poor progress in labour early, and allows timely intervention.[7,8]

When normal labour becomes abnormal labour

Different patterns of slow progress in labour may be seen and diagnosed from the partogram (Figure 4.3).

Prolonged latent phase

Until our understanding of the mechanism of the onset of labour is better, it is unlikely that we will understand why some women have a prolonged latent phase. Intervention rates are increased and augmentation of labour in women having a long latent phase does not appear to be beneficial.[9] Women with prolonged latent phase require support and adequate analgesia.

Primary dysfunctional labour

This is said to occur when the overall progress of labour is slower than the expected 1 cm per hour in a woman in whom established labour has been diagnosed. It occurs in primiparous women (26%) more commonly than multiparous women (8%).[10]

Amniotomy (artificial rupture of membranes (ARM)) can be used to shorten the length of labour (by 60–120 minutes).[11] There is however a trend towards an increase in the number of women delivered by Caesarean section. Dehydration and ketosis are associated with poor uterine contractility and intravenous fluids may help to correct this. Primary dysfunctional labour can be treated with oxytocin augmentation (although signs of obstruction must be excluded in multiparous women). (See Chapter 5 on Abnormal labour).

Secondary arrest

This is identified when normal progress in the active phase of labour ceases. It is frequently due to relative or absolute disproportion between the fetal head and the maternal pelvis. This may be because the fetal head is deflexed, e.g. OP position resulting in a wider diameter traversing the pelvis, or because of the position of the fetal head presenting a wide diameter to a narrow part of the pelvis or because the fetus is too big.

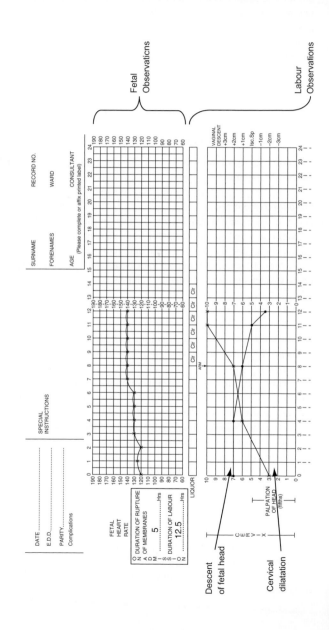

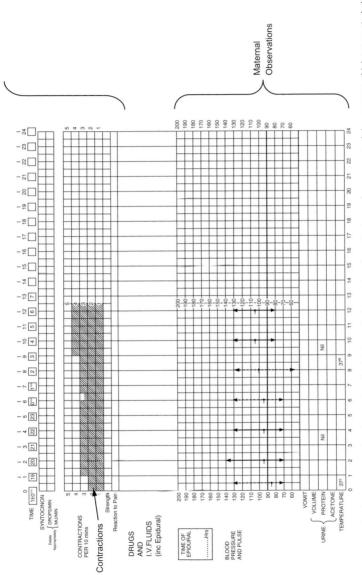

Figure 4.2 Example of a partogram showing sections for fetal monitoring, maternal monitoring and assessment of the progress of labour, particularly cervical dilatation (●) and descent of the fetal head (x), and presence of contractions (marked by bars).

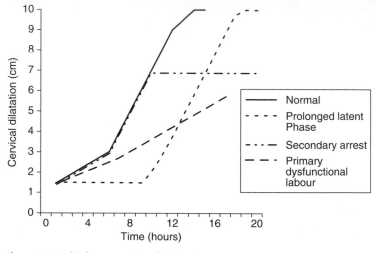

Figure 4.3 Graphical representation of abnormal patterns of labour showing prolonged latent phase, primary dysfunctional labour and secondary arrest of labour.

Emptying the woman's bladder is often a simple but useful intervention. Women with regional analgesia may be unaware that their bladder is full. In primiparous women an oxytocin infusion may overcome relative disproportion. In multiparous women secondary arrest is less common as the uterine contractility is usually better. If secondary arrest does occur in a multiparous woman there should be a high index of suspicion that this may be due to absolute, rather than relative disproportion. Under these circumstances increasing the force of contractions could lead to uterine rupture.[12] The decision to use oxytocin in a multiparous woman in active labour should be made extremely cautiously and after consultation with the consultant obstetrician on duty.

One-to-one care in labour

The concept of active management of labour consists of a package of interventions including emphasis on the correct diagnosis of the onset of labour, early amniotomy, aggressive use of oxytocin and one-to-one midwifery care in labour. The different components of the active management package have subsequently been scrutinised separately and have been mentioned above.

Continuous one-to-one care for a woman during labour has been shown to reduce the need for pain relief and lower both the incidence of Caesarean section and of operative vaginal delivery. It has also been shown that this one-to-one care does not need to be provided by a midwife but can be provided by a doula (birth assistant). The woman's confidence and feeling of control are improved.[13]

Conclusion

When managing women in labour important interventions appear to be appropriate: one-to-one support during labour, accurate diagnosis of the onset of labour, use of a partogram to identify slow progress, which in turn permits appropriate interventions including the use of amniotomy and oxytocin.

REFERENCES

1. E. A. Friedman and M. R. Sachtleben, Dysfunctional labor. *Obstet. Gynecol.*, **17** (1961), 135–48.
2. E. A. Friedman, The graphic analysis of labor. *Am. J. Obstet. Gynecol.*, **68** (1954), 1568–75.
3. E. A. Friedman, Primigravid labor. *Obstet. Gynecol.*, **6** (1955), 567–89.
4. E. A. Friedman, Labor in multiparas. *Obstet. Gynecol.*, **8** (1956), 691–703.
5. National Collaborating Centre for Women's Health (Commissioned by National Institute for Health and Clinical Excellence), *Intrapartum Care of Healthy Women and their Babies During Childbirth* (Draft Guidelines) (London: RCOG Press, 2006).
6. S. Vause, H. M. Congdon and J. G. Thornton, A randomised controlled trial of early versus delayed pushing in second stage of labour for nulliparous women with epidurals *Br. J. Obstet. Gynaecol.*, **105** (1998), 186–8.
7. R. H. Philpott and W. M. Castle, Cervicographs in the management of labour in primigravidae II. The action line and treatment of abnormal labour. *J. Obstet. Gynaecol. Br. Commonw.*, **79** (1972), 599–602.
8. World Health Organization, Partograph in management of labour. *Lancet*, **343** (1994), 1399–404.
9. D. Chelmow, S. J. Kilpatrick and R. K. Laros, Maternal and neonatal outcomes after prolonged latent phase. *Obstet. Gynecol.*, **81** (1993), 486–91.
10. E. Z. Friedman, K. R. Niswander, M. R. Sachtleben and M. Ashworth, Dysfunctional labor IX. Delivery outcome. *Am. J. Obstet. Gynecol.*, **106** (1970), 219–26.
11. W. D. Fraser, L. Turcot, I. Krauss and G. Brisson-Carrol, Amniotomy for shortening spontaneous labour. *Cochrane Database Syst. Rev.*, **2** (2005), CD000015.
12. *Confidential Enquiry into Stillbirths and Deaths in Infancy*, Fifth Annual Report (London: RCOG Press 1998).
13. J. G. Thornton and R. J. Lilford, Active management of labour: current knowledge and research issues. *BMJ*, **309** (1994), 336–9.

Abnormal labour

Jenny Myers

Introduction

Abnormal labour represents a large proportion of obstetric and anaesthetic work load on the labour ward.

Pre-term labour

Preterm labour is defined as the onset of spontaneous contractions before 37 weeks gestation. In current practice, intervention in the form of tocolysis would usually be considered in women presenting with contractions prior to 34 weeks gestation in view of the significant implications for perinatal morbidity and mortality in these cases. Preterm delivery is the leading cause of neonatal mortality. The survival rate of babies born in the developed world now ranges from 17 % for babies born at 23 weeks to over 90 % for babies born at 30 weeks. Mortality rates are directly related to both gestation and birthweight, with birth weight being a better predictor of survival after 29 weeks gestation. Multiple pregnancies are associated with poorer neonatal survival rates when compared to singleton pregnancies at the same gestation and neonatal mortality is significantly higher in male infants. In addition to neonatal mortality, prematurity is associated with significant long-term morbidity and disability. Significant ongoing motor impairment occurs in approximately 1 in 4 low-birth weight infants (<1500 g) and approximately 1 in 3 have hearing or visual impairments. Premature and low-birth weight babies are also more likely to have chronic lung disease, require hospital admission for acute illness and develop cardiovascular disease in later life.

There are a number of identifiable risk factors associated with preterm labour, which are listed below. Infection is the commonest cause of preterm labour, however, in a significant proportion of cases a cause is not identified.

- Previous preterm delivery
- Infection
- Multiple pregnancy
- Maternal medical disease
- Maternal factors such as low body mass index (BMI), smoking and poor socio-economic status
- Uterine anomalies
- Cervical incompetence secondary to congenital weakness, cone biopsy, iatrogenic damage

Obstetrics for Anaesthetists, ed. Alexander Heazell and John Clift. Published by Cambridge University Press. © Cambridge University Press 2008

Assessment of women with threatened premature labour

The management of threatened preterm labour is aimed at maximising neonatal survival by prolonging the pregnancy. The administration of corticosteroids 24–48 hours prior to delivery significantly improves perinatal morbidity and mortality; therefore in the short term tocolytic therapy aims to prolong the pregnancy for 24 hours at least. Each case must be assessed individually but in the presence of severe clinical chorioamnionitis prolongation of the pregnancy may not be beneficial to the mother or baby.

Uterine activity is assessed clinically and in the presence of persistent contractions cervical assessment is necessary. Vigilant observation to detect infection is very important and the presence of tachycardia, pyrexia, uterine tenderness, purulent vaginal discharge, raised inflammatory markers or Cardiotocograph (CTG) changes may all indicate chorioamnionitis. Continuous fetal monitoring should only be used in situations where abnormalities would justify iatrogenic delivery; this needs to be carefully assessed in cases of extreme prematurity.

> The use of regional analgesia is contraindicated in patients with untreated sepsis due to the risk of meningitis and extradural abscess. Once antibiotics have been commenced an assessment of the risks and benefits should be made.

Treatment options

The decision to attempt to arrest preterm labour with tocolytic therapy is dependent on the following factors:

- Gestation
- Maternal and fetal condition
- Progress of labour i.e. labour may be too advanced to attempt tocolysis

  Tocolytic therapy in established preterm labour has a poor efficacy. The current treatment options include:
- Sublingual nifedipine: 10 mg every 15 minutes up to 4 doses, followed by an oral maintenance regime
- PR indomethacin: 100 mg bd for up to 48 hours (<32 weeks only)
- Atosiban (oxytocin receptor antagonist) IV infusion for up to 24 hours

> - If labour proceeds, delivery is frequently rapid and often does not require analgesia
> - Regional analgesia may be beneficial in some situations such as malpresentation and multiple pregnancy
> - If operative delivery is indicated, in the absence of significant maternal infection, regional analgesia would be the anaesthesia of choice

Abnormal first stage of labour – slow progress in labour

The progress of normal labour is discussed in Chapter 4. Deviation from this normal progress is termed 'delay in the first stage' or 'failure to progress' and can be broadly classified into prolonged latent phase, primary dysfunctional labour and secondary arrest (see Figure 5.1).

Prolonged latent phase is difficult to define as the onset is difficult to determine accurately. Support, explanation and analgesia are necessary in these cases to avoid unnecessary intervention, which is associated with higher operative delivery rates.

Primary dysfunctional labour was defined by Friedman as active phase progress of less than 1 cm per hour.[1] In practice, dysfunctional labour is diagnosed in women thought to be in the active stage of labour, (i.e. >3–4 cm dilated) who have not made adequate progress on two or more successive vaginal examinations 4 hours apart. Secondary arrest is defined as the cessation of cervical dilatation following a normal portion of active phase cervical dilatation. Secondary arrest is most likely to be associated with cephalo-pelvic disproportion.

Intervention for slow progress in labour

It is common to think of labour in terms of powers, passages and the passenger. As there is little the clinician can do to manipulate the latter two of these variables, the only remaining option is to attempt to increase the powers using oxytocin.

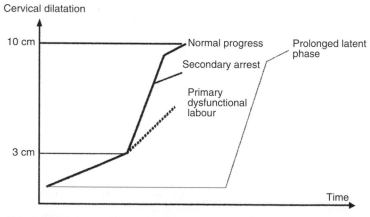

Figure 5.1 Graphical representation of abnormal patterns of labour showing prolonged latent phase, primary dysfunctional labour and secondary arrest of labour.

In women in active labour (>3 cm dilated) with intact amniotic membranes, amniotomy should always be performed prior to the use of oxytocics. Oxytocin is used commonly in abnormal labour and effectively increases uterine activity and causes cervical dilatation; however, this does not necessarily translate into uncomplicated vaginal delivery. Cardiotocograph abnormalities and consequent fetal blood sampling, and instrumental delivery are all very common in these mothers. Caesarean delivery rates have been shown to be tenfold greater in women with secondary arrest despite further cervical dilatation following oxytocin,[2] and randomised controlled trials have not been able to show the expected benefit of oxytocin.[3,4] Oxytocin should be used cautiously in multiparous women in view of the risk of uterine rupture and should only be used after clinical assessment by a senior obstetrician.

> Women with slow progress in the first stage of labour will often benefit from epidural analgesia, especially if oxytocin is used as augmented contractions are more painful than spontaneous contractions.

Use of oxytocin is associated with:
- Uterine hyperstimulation
- Fetal distress
- Instrumental/operative delivery

Uterine hyperstimulation

Uterine hyperstimulation is a common side effect of oxytocin administration and this is the reason for the incremental regime used to accelerate or induce labour. Ideally contractions should occur regularly at a frequency of 3–5 every 10 minutes with a rest phase between contractions. Contractions occurring more frequently or without an appropriate rest phase may result in fetal heart rate abnormalities (See Figure 5.2). Fetal heart rate abnormalities can usually be corrected by discontinuing or reducing the dose of oxytocin. A fetal blood sample may need to be performed and in some cases early delivery by Caesarean section is indicated. Iatrogenic uterine hyperstimulation can be treated by administration of subcutaneous terbutaline 250 µg), sublingual glyceryl trinitrate (0.5 mg) or inhaled salbutamol (5 mg).

Abnormal second stage of labour

Delay in the second stage is usually defined as failure to deliver following an active second stage of 1 hour. There are a number of factors that influence the length of the second stage including parity, uterine activity, position of the fetal head, analgesia and maternal effort.

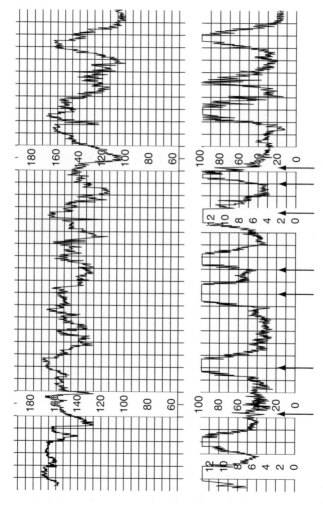

Figure 5.2 Cardiotocograph demonstrating uterine hyperstimulation, with uterine activity, 5 contractions (marked with arrows) in 10 minutes (marked by lines). (Reproduced with permission from J. Gardosi, T. Vanner, L. Chadwick, and M. Terret – CTG Tutor, PRAM, 1996. Perinatal Institute. www.pi.nhs.uk/ctg.)

Some of these factors can be optimised by the obstetrician and midwife to increase the chance of a spontaneous vaginal delivery or uncomplicated instrumental delivery. These include:

- A passive second stage to allow descent of the fetal head – for women with epidural analgesia this can be up to 2 hours in the presence of a normal CTG
- Oxytocin should be considered in the presence of inadequate uterine contractions (used with extreme caution in multiparous patients)
- Encouragement is very important and the mother should be given the opportunity to push in different positions if possible
- Bladder catheterisation aids descent of the presenting part
- Manual rotation of an occipito-transverse (OT) or occipito-posterior (OP) position of the fetal head may be possible in some instances and facilitate a normal delivery (usually only possible in the presence of adequate analgesia)

> Prolonged second stage of labour is an indication for instrumental vaginal delivery. If the presenting part is high or the fetal position is OP or OT instrumental vaginal delivery should be attempted in the operating theatre under adequate anaesthesia for Caesarean section, which is required for unsuccessful vaginal delivery.

Malpresentations and malpositions

Abnormal progress in the first and second stage of labour is associated with fetal malpresentations and malpositions. Cervical dilatation and descent of the presenting part is dependent upon the application of the presenting part to the cervix. Breech presentation is associated with prolonged first stage of labour which should be managed with caution (see Assisted vaginal breech delivery in Chapter 8).

Malpositions, such as OP and OT positions are associated with prolonged first and second stages of labour. These are diagnosed on vaginal examination by palpation of the cranial sutures. The delay results from the requirement of the fetal head to rotate to an occipito-anterior (OA) position for delivery to occur in the majority of cases; this may be facilitated by augmentation of labour with oxytocin.

> There is an association, but no evidence of causation, between epidural analgesia and the OP position. The association is probably because of the increased analgesic requirements.

Brow presentation, in which the fetal forehead presents first cannot deliver vaginally and must be delivered by Caesarean section (Figure 5.3A). Face presentation, in which the fetal face presents first (Figure 5.3B), can deliver vaginally if the chin is anterior (mento-anterior). Mento-posterior positions (chin posterior) cannot deliver vaginally and must be delivered by Caesarean section.

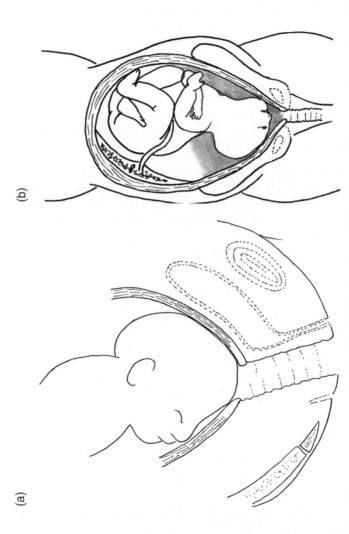

Figure 5.3 Malpresentations. A) Brow presentation, note the diameter of the fetal head is too large to enter the maternal pelvis – hence operative delivery is required. B) Face presentation – if the fetal chin (mentum) is anterior the baby can be delivered vaginally.

Epidural analgesia is ideal for malpresentations attempting a vaginal delivery because there is an increase in:
- Duration of labour
- Pain during labour
- Incidence of instrumental and operative delivery

Consequently, the position of the fetus must be carefully assessed before commencing augmentation of labour. Augmentation of labour in positions unable to deliver vaginally is associated with uterine rupture. Brow and mento-posterior positions should not receive oxytocin.

Abnormal third stage of labour – retained placenta

Third stage of labour is completed following delivery of the placenta and a retained placenta has been described as failure to deliver the placenta 30–60 minutes following delivery of the baby. Retained placenta occurs in 0.5–1% of deliveries and occurs more commonly in women with a history of retained placenta, scarring of the uterus, chorioamnionitis and at early gestations.[5]

Postpartum haemorrhage is associated with retained placenta and requires adequate resuscitation. Therefore, all women with a retained placenta should be cannulated and have a full blood count (FBC) and group and save sample obtained prior to an attempt at removal. Adequate analgesia is essential as manual removal of the placenta is very uncomfortable for the mother.

Intervention

Manual removal of the placenta should be conducted under sterile conditions with adequate analgesia. Once the obstetrician has removed the placenta and checked that the uterine cavity is empty, an infusion of oxytocin should be commenced (40 iu over 4 hours). Prophylactic broad-spectrum intravenous antibiotics should also be given intraoperatively.

Implications of retained placenta
- The obstetrician removes the placenta in the operating theatre
- FBC, group and save should be done
- Assessment for hypovolaemia should be made and adequate resuscitation be given prior to administration of anaesthesia.
- Regional anaesthesia is the anaesthesia of choice (epidural if *in situ* or spinal)
- Oxytocin 5 iu slow bolus should be given, and an infusion of 10 iu/hr should be considered
- Broad-spectrum antibiotics should be given

Morbid placental adherence (placenta accreta)

Placenta accreta is suspected if during removal of the placenta a plane of cleavage cannot identified. The degree of adherence is described according to the level of invasion through the uterine wall and is usually associated with uterine scarring.

- Accreta – adherent to the myometrium
- Increta – invasion into the myometrium
- Percreta – penetrates through the myometrium to the serosal surface

Senior obstetric and anaesthetic input is vital in suspected cases of placenta accreta and maternal mortality is lower if an aggressive operative approach is instituted, i.e. hysterectomy.[6] Some successful conservative approaches have been reported, including expectant management with/without methotrexate, blunt dissection and curettage and conservative surgery involving ligation of the uterine vessels. These are associated with haemorrhage, sepsis and persistent placental retention and should only be considered where preservation of fertility is of overriding importance.

Retained placenta is a cause of major obstetric haemorrhage.

Emergencies in labour – cord prolapse, shoulder dystocia

Cord prolapse

Prolapse of the umbilical cord occurs in 1–2/1000 deliveries and is associated with breech presentation, multiple pregnancy, prematurity and transverse lie. Spontaneous or artificial rupture of the membranes with a high head is a common cause of cord prolapse. Cord prolapse is an obstetric emergency but with prompt intervention a good neonatal outcome can be expected.

Management

The management of cord prolapse involves elevation of the presenting part to reduce cord compression and prompt delivery. Elevation of the presenting part can be achieved by turning the mother onto 'all fours', digital elevation of the presenting part or rapid filling of the bladder with 500 ml of normal saline (effective in cases of cord prolapse that do not occur on the delivery unit). If a quick and safe vaginal delivery is not possible, an emergency Caesarean section should be performed. Measures employed to elevate the presenting part should continue during transfer to the operating theatre and preparation for surgery.

Anaesthetic implications:
- Intrauterine resuscitation should be commenced immediately (see below)
- Cord prolapse is an indication for category 1 Caesarean section if there is fetal distress
- General or spinal anaesthesia should be administered as quickly as possible whilst considering the safety of the mother and condition of the fetus; the decision to delivery interval should be <30 minutes
- If there are no signs of fetal distress, spinal anaesthesia or epidural 'top-up' could be administered whilst continuously monitoring the fetal heart
- There should be early recourse to general anaesthesia if there is fetal distress or multiple attempts at regional anaesthesia

Intrauterine resuscitation for cord prolapse:
- Do not handle the umbilical cord
- Alter maternal position: left lateral, head-down, or head-down knee-to-chest position. Manually displace presenting part.
- Intravenous fluids
- Oxygen
- Tocolysis: terbutaline 250 µg sc
- Continuous fetal monitoring
- Fill bladder with 500 ml normal saline if operating theatre not immediately available

Shoulder dystocia

Shoulder dystocia is a very serious obstetric emergency and in current obstetric practice is a significant cause of perinatal morbidity and mortality; consequently it is a leading cause of litigation claims. The commonest fetal injuries include brachial plexus damage, clavicular fractures and, in severe cases, long-term complications arising from fetal asphyxia may occur.

Shoulder dystocia is broadly defined as difficulty in delivering the shoulders following delivery of the head; however, a true dystocia requires manoeuvres to disimpact the shoulders and facilitate delivery.

Risk factors

One of the most important challenges regarding shoulder dystocia is that it is unpredictable. There are, however, a number of risk factors that should alert obstetricians and midwives to the possibility of a difficult delivery.

Antenatal:
- Maternal diabetes
- Estimated fetal weight >4500 g – there is a 10–20%[7] error when predicting fetal weight by ultrasound

- Maternal weight and height – the risk of shoulder dystocia is increased with maternal height, excessive weight gain in pregnancy and BMI
- Prior macrosomic infant (> 4500 g)
- Previous shoulder dystocia – recurrence risk is controversial as the data are contradictory[8,9]

In labour:
- Slow progress in the first stage of labour
- Delay in second stage particularly in multiparous women
- May require instrumental delivery

Mechanism of shoulder delivery
After delivery of the head, spontaneous external rotation returns the head to its perpendicular relationship to the shoulders, which are usually in the oblique position. Maternal effort and uterine propulsion will normally drive the anterior shoulder under the symphysis. If the shoulders fail to rotate to the oblique axis and remain in the antero-posterior position expulsive force will drive the anterior shoulder against the symphysis causing impaction.

Management
Modern labour ward 'drills' include the management of severe shoulder dystocia and all health professionals involved in labour ward care should be aware of these procedures. For mothers where a difficult delivery of the shoulders is anticipated, appropriate senior medical staff should be present at delivery.

- Call for **help** – this should include senior midwives, senior obstetric staff and a paediatrician. Initialisation of effective preliminary measures requires at least four people and therefore everyone close by can be useful.
- Perform an **episiotomy** – this does not help delivery of the shoulders but allows more room for manoeuvres to be performed.
- **McRoberts postion** – flexion of hips and knees or 'knees-to-chest' position. This requires the back of the bed to be lowered and two individuals to flex and hold each leg.
- **Suprapubic pressure** – this should be applied from the side of the bed nearest the fetus' back.
- **Manoeuvres**
  - Delivery of the **posterior arm** – this allows the anterior shoulder to disimpact
  - **Woodscrew manoeuvre** – this involves rotation of the shoulders to bring the posterior shoulder to the anterior position and can be attempted in either direction
- **Symphysiotomy** – this is only used as a last resort in very severe cases and involves division of the symphysis ligaments using a scalpel. This can be done following infiltration with local anaesthetic.

- **Zavanelli manoeuvre** has been described to replace the head in the vagina so that a Caesarean section may be performed. In practice this is very difficult and rarely attempted in modern obstetrics.

Following a delivery involving a shoulder dystocia appropriate debriefing and counselling for the family is essential. Accurate documentation of timings, the health professionals involved and the procedures necessary to facilitate delivery is also vital.

Anaesthetic implications:
- Disimpaction procedures are much easier if anaesthesia has been given to the mother
- General anaesthesia is usually the best choice as anaesthesia is required immediately
- Shoulder dystocia is associated with postpartum haemorrhage

REFERENCES

1. E. Friedman, Dysfunctional labour. *Obstet. Gynecol.*, **17**:2 (1961), 135–8.
2. L. D. Cardozo, D. M. Gibb, J. W. Studd, R. V. Vasant and D. J. Cooper, Predictive value of cervimetric labour patterns in primigravidae. *Br. J. Obstet. Gynaecol.*, **89**:1 (1982), 33–8.
3. H. Cammu and E. Van Eeckhout, A randomised controlled trial of early versus delayed use of amniotomy and oxytocin infusion in nulliparous labour. *Br. J. Obstet. Gynaecol.*, **103**:4 (1996), 313–8.
4. F. D. Frigoletto, Jr, E. Lieberman, J. M. Lang *et al.*, A clinical trial of active management of labor. *N. Engl. J. Med.*, **333**:12 (1995), 745–50.
5. B. Sorbe, Active pharmacologic management of the third stage of labor. A comparison of oxytocin and ergometrine. *Obstet. Gynecol.*, **52**:6 (1978), 694–7.
6. J. A. Read, D. B. Cotton and F. C. Miller, Placenta accreta: changing clinical aspects and outcome. *Obstet. Gynecol.*, **56**:1 (1980), 31–4.
7. G. I. Hirata, A. L. Medearis, J. Horenstein, M. B. Bear and L. D. Platt, Ultrasonographic estimation of fetal weight in the clinically macrosomic fetus. *Am. J. Obstet. Gynecol.*, **162**:1 (1990), 238–42.
8. T. F. Baskett and A. C. Allen, Perinatal implications of shoulder dystocia. *Obstet. Gynecol.*, **86**:1 (1995), 14–17.
9. D. F. Lewis, R. C. Raymond, M. B. Perkins, G. G. Brooks and A. R. Heymann, Recurrence rate of shoulder dystocia. *Am. J. Obstet. Gynecol.*, **172**:5 (1995), 1369–71.

FURTHER READING

D. M. Levy, Anaesthesia for Caesarean section. *Continuing Education in Anaesthesia, Critical Care and Pain*, **1** (2001), 171–6.
C. Thomas and T. Madej, Obstetric emergencies and the anaesthetist. *Continuing Education in Anaesthesia, Critical Care and Pain* **2** (2002), 174–7.

Fetal monitoring

Justine Nugent

Introduction

Electronic fetal monitoring (EFM) describes the use of electronic detection of the fetal heart rate for the evaluation of fetal well being. It was first introduced into the UK in the 1970s before its clinical effectiveness had been fully evaluated. The aim of EFM was to "prevent harm" and improve birth outcomes by detecting fetal hypoxia before it led to death and disability. The current prevalence rates for perinatal mortality and cerebral palsy are 8 and 1.1 per 1000 live births respectively, the prevalence for those attributable to an intrapartum event are 0.8 and 0.1 per 1000 births respectively.[1]

EFM is primarily a screening test. It is a highly sensitive test detecting a disease with a low prevalence. It has a high false-positive rate and poor positive predictive value. An improvement in specificity would decrease the sensitivity but would make the test falsely reassuring, reducing the detection of potentially compromised babies.

Monitoring low- and high-risk pregnancies

Intermittent auscultation

The fetal heart rate (FHR) is monitored intermittently using a hand-held Doppler USS device or Pinard Stethoscope (Figure 6.1). In the active stages of labour, intermittent auscultation should occur after a contraction for a minimum of 60 seconds, every 15 minutes during the first stage and every 5 minutes in the second stage of labour.

> **Intermittent auscultation** is recommended for monitoring fetal well being during normal labour provided the woman is healthy and the pregnancy is uncomplicated.

Intermittent auscultation compared to continuous EFM

There have been several systematic reviews comparing these two forms of monitoring.[2,3] When compared with intermittent auscultation, continuous fetal monitoring is associated with:

- an increase in operative delivery rates – both Caesarean section and instrumental deliveries
- a reduction in neonatal seizures but there was no significant difference in either Apgar scores or neonatal intensive care admissions

Obstetrics for Anaesthetists, ed. Alexander Heazell and John Clift. Published by Cambridge University Press. © Cambridge University Press 2008

(a)

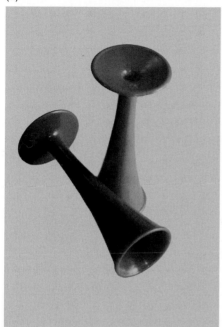

(b)

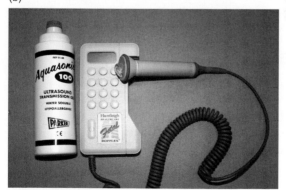

Figure 6.1 Instruments used for auscultation of the fetal heart (a) Pinard Stethoscope (b) Hand-held Doppler device. These may both be used for intermittent fetal heart auscultation during labour.

Table 6.1 Antenatal and intrapartum factors indicating a need for continuous electronic fetal monitoring

Antenatal factors

Maternal	**Fetal**
Hypertension/Pre-eclampsia	Small fetus/intrauterine growth restriction
Diabetes mellitus	Premature (< 37 weeks)
Antepartum haemorrhage	Multiple pregnancy
Cardiac disease	Breech presentation
Renal disease	Previous intrauterine fetal death
Connective tissue disorder	
Hyperthyroidism	

Intrapartum factors

Maternal	**Fetal**	**Labour**
Vaginal bleeding in labour	Meconium-stained liquor	Previous Caesarean section
Intrauterine infection	Suspicious FHR on auscultation	Prolonged rupture of membranes
Epidural analgesia	Post-term pregnancy	Induction of labour
		Labour augmented with oxytocin

Continuous fetal monitoring was not associated with any demonstrable reduction in perinatal mortality. However, this finding should be interpreted with caution; when all trials comparing intermittent auscultation with continuous EFM are combined together they are still significantly underpowered to detect a difference in perinatal mortality. Continuous EFM is indicated for maternal or fetal reasons that may be grouped into antenatal or intrapartum factors (Table 6.1). These include conditions that pre-dispose to fetal hypoxia or result from interventions in normal labour.

Continuous EFM is recommended for high-risk pregnancies where there is an increased risk of perinatal death, cerebral palsy or neonatal encephalopathy.

Electronic fetal monitoring

The **fetal heart rate** (FHR) trace or **cardiotocograph** (CTG) has five recognisable features: uterine activity, baseline FHR, baseline variability, accelerations and decelerations. In the UK the majority of CTGs are recorded at 1 cm/min, which is reflected in the CTG paper with intersections at 1 and 10 minute intervals. Continuous fetal monitoring can be undertaken via an abdominal Doppler

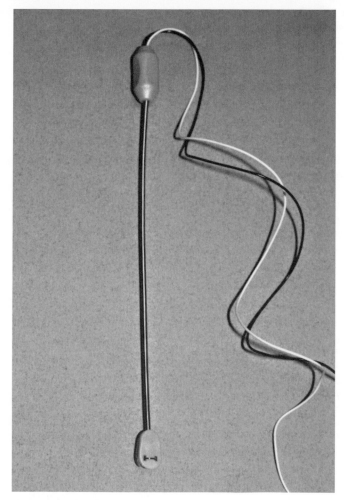

Figure 6.2 Fetal scalp electrode – used when heart rate monitoring via a transabdominal ultrasound transducer is poor due to maternal habitus, maternal mobility, or fetal position.

ultrasound transducer or via a fetal scalp electrode (Figure 6.2), which directly records fetal cardiac electrical activity.

Description of terms

Uterine activity Unless this is recorded using an intrauterine pressure catheter this cannot give a measure of 'strength' of a contraction. Frequency of contractions can be assessed, and is normally described as the average number of contractions in 10 minutes.

Baseline FHR is the mean level of the fetal heart rate. Normal FHR is 110–160 bpm. Fetal *bradycardia* is defined as < 100 bpm and a fetal *tachycardia* > 160 bpm.

Baseline variability describes the minor fluctuations in baseline heart rate or the bandwidth or 'wiggliness' of the trace. Normal baseline variability is > 5 bpm and abnormal < 5 bpm for > 45 minutes.

Accelerations are transient increases in the FHR of > 15 bpm for > 15 seconds.

Decelerations describe a decrease of the FHR of > 15 bpm from the baseline FHR for > 15 seconds. Decelerations are further classified into *early, late, variable* and *prolonged*.

Early decelerations are the periodic slowing of the FHR that commences at the start of the contraction and returns to baseline at the end of the contraction (Figure 6.3).

Mechanism: Early decelerations are due to head compression and are common in the late first stage and second stage of labour. Isolated early decelerations do not suggest hypoxaemia.

Late decelerations are the slowing of the FHR that commences mid to late contraction, the lowest point (nadir) is > 20 seconds from the peak of the contraction and ending after the contraction (Figure 6.4).

Mechanism: During labour, the blood supply to the placenta is interrupted during a uterine contraction and a healthy fetus derives oxygen from the retro-placental pool of blood. If the oxygen in the retro-placental pool of maternal blood is insufficient then the FHR slows via fetal chemoreceptor mechanisms. The FHR recovers once perfusion to the retro-placental bed and therefore the oxygen supply to the fetus is restored.

Variable decelerations are rapid in onset and recovery; they are variable in terms of shape, size and timing in the contraction cycle.

Mechanism: Variable decelerations are usually due to cord compression. When the cord is compressed, the thin-walled vein is occluded first. Blood continues to leave the fetus via the more robust arteries causing hypotension, which in turn increases the heart rate. The umbilical arteries are then occluded resulting in a relative hypertension, which causes a fall in heart rate via the baroreceptor mechanism. When the pressure on the cord is released, the artery opens first, allowing blood again to leave the fetus causing a fall in blood pressure and an increase in FHR above the baseline. During uterine relaxation, the vein opens and the perfusion to and from the fetus is re-established and the FHR returns to normal (Figure 6.5).

Atypical variable decelerations are variable decelerations with any of the additional features listed below:

- Loss of rise in baseline before or after the deceleration
- Slow return of fetal heart to the baseline after the contraction

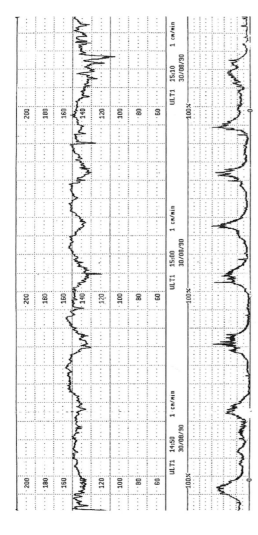

Figure 6.3 Cardiotocograph showing early decelerations. (Reproduced from D. Gibb and S. Arulkumaran, *Fetal Monitoring in Practice*, 2nd edn, Butterworth–Heinemann, London, 1997 with permission from Elsevier.)

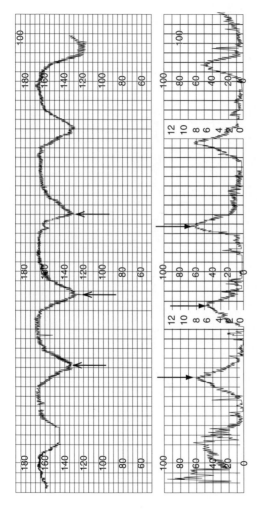

Figure 6.4 Cardiotocograph showing late decelerations. The nadir of the deceleration (open arrows) occurs after peak of the contraction (closed arrows) (Reproduced from J. Gardosi, T. Vanner, L. Vanner, L. Chadwick and M. Terret – CTG Tutor, PRAM, 1996. Perinatal Institute. www.pi.nhs.uk/ctg.)

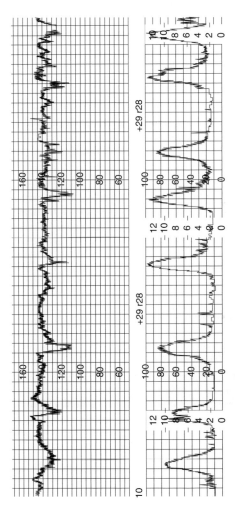

Figure 6.5 Cardiotocograph showing variable decelerations (Reproduced from J. Gardosi, T. Vanner, L. Chadwick and M. Terret – CTG Tutor, PRAM, 1996. Perinatal Institute. www.pi.nhs.uk/ctg.)

- Prolonged rise in baseline following the deceleration
- Biphasic deceleration
- Loss of variability during the deceleration
- Continuation of baseline at lower level

These features are associated with an increased risk of adverse neonatal outcome.

Mechanism: A well grown baby can tolerate cord compression for a certain length of time; after that the FHR trace will begin to show signs of developing hypoxia.

A *prolonged deceleration* is a sudden decrease in the FHR below its baseline that lasts at least 60–90 seconds. These decelerations become pathological if they last more than 3 minutes.

Additional feature of CTGs

Sinusoidal pattern describes a smooth, regular oscillation of the baseline variability resembling a sine wave with an amplitude of 5–15 bpm and a frequency of 3–5 cycles per minutes (Figure 6.6).[4] In uncompromised fetuses a sinusoidal pattern for < 10 minutes does not appear to be associated with a poor outcome. However, a prolonged sinusoidal trace has been associated with fetal anaemia or hypoxia and a poor neonatal outcome. Therefore, if this pattern develops in labour a fetal maternal haemorrhage should be considered.

Fetal hypoxia

Hypoxia can develop gradually or suddenly during labour as a result of:

- Occlusion of the umbilical cord
- Decreased perfusion of the placental bed
- Inadequate retro-placental pool for oxygen exchange during a contraction

Hypoxia is unlikely to develop in the absence of FHR decelerations. The presence of decelerations without a rise in baseline heart rate or a reduction in baseline variability, i.e. still reactive, is called the stress period and the fetus is compensating. Initially the fetus may respond to the inadequate supply of oxygen by increasing its cardiac output by increasing its heart rate, which may be associated with a reduction in accelerations.

As the hypoxia worsens, the autonomic nervous system is affected; in addition to the increase in the FHR there is also a gradual reduction in baseline variability. Once the fetus has achieved its maximum baseline heart rate and the baseline variability falls to < 5 bpm, the fetus moves from the stress to the distress period. Later the CTG may show variable decelerations with severe hypoxic features i.e. loss of baseline variability and a baseline tachycardia. This distress stage indicates that the fetus may be or will soon become hypoxaemic or acidaemic. Fetal blood sampling should be performed at this stage (see later for more details). If the

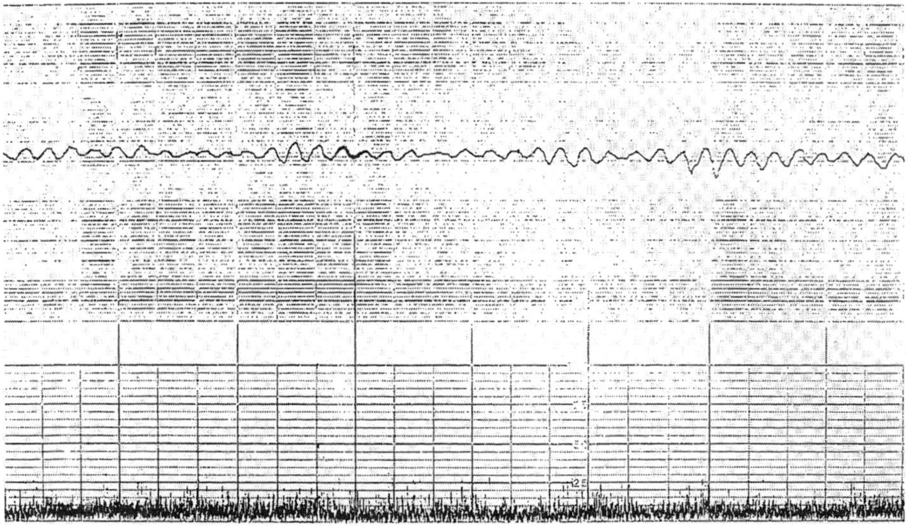

Figure 6.6 Cardiotocograph showing a sinusoidal trace (Reproduced from D. Gibb and S. Arulkumaran, *Fetal Monitoring in Practice*, 2nd edn, Butterworth-Heinemann, London, 1997 with permission from Elsevier.)

Table 6.2 The overall classification of CTG by assessment of individual features of the trace

Feature	Baseline (bpm)	Variability (bpm)	Decelerations	Accelerations
Reassuring	110–160	> 5	None	Present
Non-reassuring	100–109 161–180	< 5 for > 40 min but < 90 min	Early Variable Single prolonged > 3 min	The absence of accelerations with an otherwise normal CTG is
Abnormal	< 100 > 180 Sinusoidal > 10 min	< 5 for > 90 min	Atypical variable Late Single prolonged deceleration > 3 min	of uncertain significance

Adapted from *The Use and Interpretation of Cardiotocography in Intrapartum Fetal Surveillance – Evidence-based Clinical Guideline 8.*[5]

situation is ignored, the FHR declines to a terminal bradycardia. This is also called the distress to death period and is relatively short, lasting between 20 and 60 minutes.

A fetus with *chronic hypoxia* prior to the onset of labour, which may occur in growth-restricted fetuses, would have a trace with a baseline variability of < 5 bpm and exhibit shallow decelerations (< 15 bpm from the baseline heart rate) with the onset of contractions. Although these shallow decelerations do not meet traditional definitions, this feature along with the loss of baseline variability is very ominous and there may be a sudden fetal bradycardia and fetal demise (within 1–2 hours).

The National Institute for Health and Clinical Excellence guidelines on electronic fetal monitoring (2001)[5] recommend that a CTG or FHR trace is classified into one of three groups: normal, suspicious or pathological based on the presence of reassuring and non-reassuring features; these features are defined in Table 6.2.

A normal CTG will have normal baseline of 110–150 bpm, good variability of > 5 bpm, accelerations and no decelerations. Accelerations and a normal baseline variability are the hallmarks of fetal health (Figure 6.7).

Suspicious CTG

Definition
A suspicious CTG has one non-reassuring feature and the remainder of the features are all reassuring.

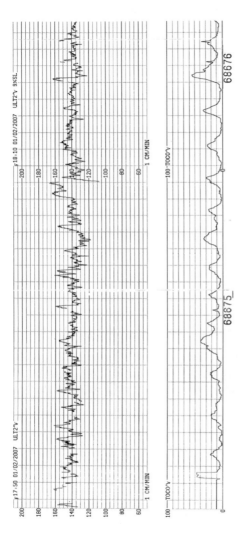

Figure 6.7 A normal cardiotocography trace: note the normal baseline heart rate, the fetal heart variability, the presence of accelerations and absence of decelerations.

Action

In cases where the CTG falls into the suspicious category conservative measures should be employed. These include:

- Correcting maternal hypovolaemia and/or hypotension
- Diminishing the uterine activity, especially if excessive, by stopping oxytocin and considering tocolysis e.g. 250 μg subcutaneous terbutaline
- Improve maternal oxygenation – *this should not be used for more than a few minutes unless there is low maternal saturation* as there is no evidence to suggest benefit and there is a suggestion that it might be detrimental
- Excluding a complication indicating emergency delivery such as abruption, cord prolapse, chorioamnionitis and scar dehiscence
- Continuously monitoring the fetus and the trace observed for the development of pathological features

  The presence of persistent suspicious features is an indication for fetal blood sampling.

  The mother should be informed of the concerns and be involved in the management plan.

Pathological CTG

Definition

A pathological CTG has two or more non-reassuring features and one or more abnormal changes.

Action

Conservative methods should be employed, as above, if they have not been already. Fetal blood sampling (FBS) is also indicated. If FBS is inappropriate/not possible (e.g. cervix < 3 cm dilated) or the result suggests hypoxia, delivery should be expedited.

Prolonged fetal bradycardia

Acute hypoxia produces a prolonged fetal bradycardia. This can occur as a result of:

- Placental abruption
- Cord prolapse
- Scar dehiscence or rupture

  A fetal bradycardia as a result of any of the above needs immediate delivery.

  In the absence of any of the above conditions, reversible causes can be sought and simple measures can be employed to try and restore the FHR. Reversible causes include:

- Epidural top-up causing maternal hypotension
- Supine hypotension e.g. following a vaginal examination

- Vagal stimulus e.g. vomiting
- Uterine hyperstimulation

Measures for intrauterine resuscitation to try and restore FHR include:
- Adjusting maternal position to left lateral
- Stopping oxytocin
- Hydration
- Oxygen via a face-mask

Hypoxia and acidosis will occur if the bradycardia persists beyond 10 minutes in a healthy fetus. If no action is taken and the bradycardia is allowed to persist, fetal demise or a poor neonatal outcome will result. Whilst anxiously waiting for the FHR to return to normal, the clinical situation needs to be taken into account. In a previously uncompromised fetus, delivery should be expedited after 10 minutes and in a compromised fetus after 6 minutes. Examples of a compromised fetus include:
- Abnormal FHR trace immediately prior to the bradycardia
- A growth-restricted fetus
- Oligohydramnios or thick meconium-stained liquor

   Fetal blood sampling has no role in acute events e.g. as in a prolonged deceleration when the baby should be delivered.

- Prolonged fetal bradycardia requires delivery immediately
- If not deliverable by immediate instrumental delivery, will need category 1 Caesarean section, which will usually require a general anaesthetic

Fetal blood sampling

Fetal blood sampling (FBS) is used to identify compromised fetuses that need immediate delivery from those that are fine. It is performed in the left lateral or lithotomy position. The cervix needs to be at least 2–3 cm dilated and an amnioscope is inserted into the vagina and used to visualise the fetal head (Figure 6.8). The scalp is cleaned and a small 'scratch' is made. A microtube is filled with blood, approximately 25 µl, and the pH and base excess of this capillary sample determined.

- A FBS pH > 7.25 is reassuring
  - Repeated in one hour if the FHR abnormalities persist
- pH between 7.21–7.24
  - Repeat FBS within 30 minutes
- pH ≤ 7.20
  - Delivery is indicated

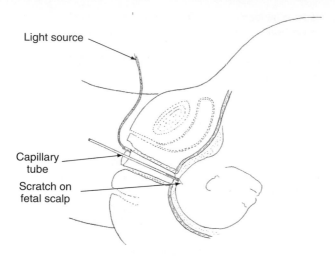

Figure 6.8 Diagram representing fetal blood sampling. An amnioscope is inserted into the vagina enabling visualisation of the fetal head, a small scratch on the fetal scalp is made with a sharp blade, and blood collected using a microtube.

> Delivery for fetal scalp pH < 7.20 requires a decision to delivery interval < 30 minutes (category 1 Caesarean section).

pH < 7.20 is two standard deviations below the mean fetal pH and was chosen to prevent an umbilical arterial pH of < 7.00 at delivery. An umbilical arterial pH of < 7.00 is associated with both short-and long-term complications for the neonate including cerebral palsy if the Apgar score at 5 minutes is also < 7. A metabolic acidosis or a 'base excess of > −12 mmol/l' represents a switch to anaerobic metabolism and is also a marker of moderate to severe morbidity.

Contraindications to FBS include:

- Maternal viral infections – HIV, hepatitis and herpes simplex virus to avoid transmission to the baby
- Maternal clotting disorders – haemophilia A, immune thrombocytopenia (ITP)
- Premature babies (< 34 weeks) – use of FBS in the presence of abnormal FHR pattern may be associated with an increase in adverse neonatal outcome

When fetal distress is **suspected** (FBS is contraindicated or is not possible) or **confirmed** (a scalp pH < 7.20 or persistent fetal bradycardia) the aim is rapid delivery of the baby. This should be accomplished as fast as possible without endangering the condition of the mother. The American College of Obstetricians and Gynaecologists (ACOG) recommends delivery of the infant within 30 minutes and this has been accepted as the standard.[6] Evidence to support this is weak and inconclusive.[5] In some instances e.g. placental abruption a decision to delivery interval of 30 minutes would be too long and in others, a delivery interval exceeding 30 minutes may not adversely affect neonatal outcome.

Additional tests of fetal surveillance

There is a need for a monitoring system with a high specificity and sensitivity for detecting fetal acidosis and allowing timely and appropriate intervention without putting the fetus at risk. Currently, systems being researched include fetal ECG analysis and fetal oxygen saturation monitoring.

Stimulation tests

An alternative method of assessment of a fetus at risk is to see if it is possible to provoke an acceleration in response to a stimuli. Accelerations during FBS or at the time of a vaginal examination are associated with a non-acidotic pH value.[7,8,9] To avoid the need for a vaginal examination, transabdominal vibro-acoustic stimulation has also been studied and shown good correlation with pH. However, babies with respiratory acidosis will also respond with accelerations and non-responders are not all acidotic.

Fetal ECG analysis

As in adult life, the fetal ECG changes with hypoxia. Fetal ECG analysis uses a fetal scalp electrode placed vaginally and uses either:

- ST waveform – in hypoxia, peaked T-wave and elevation of ST segment. Use of this with EFM significantly reduced the number of operative deliveries and there was a trend towards a reduction in FBS, but this was not significant.[10]
- PR-RR (FHR) interval – normally there is an inverse relationship between PR interval and FHR; in hypoxia this changes. PR-RR (FHR) interval in combination with EFM failed to show any benefit.[11]
- T/QRS ratio – normal < 0.25 and > 0.5 in hypoxia. T/QRS ratio with EFM had a poorer sensitivity for a pH < 7.20 than EFM alone.[12]

Fetal pulse oximetry

Oxygen saturation systems have been adapted for use in the fetus in labour. Studies have reported ease of use of the sensors and equipment but rates of adequate recording of only 70–80%. When a cut-off for normal oxygen saturation of $> 30\%$ is used, pulse oximetry has a sensitivity of 94% for a pH < 7.13 and a poor specificity (38% for pH of < 7.13).[13]

Additional notes

Meconium-stained liquor

Meconium-stained liquor is associated with increased morbidity and mortality in babies. The passage of meconium in utero occurs in 12–15% of all fetuses. Meconium-stained liquor is rare in preterm infants (< 5%), but is increasingly common in infants > 37 weeks' gestation and occurs in up to 50% of post mature (42 weeks). The incidence of meconium aspiration syndrome (MAS) when there has been meconium-stained liquor is between 1% and 5%. The severity of MAS is linked to fetal asphyxia and has a mortality rate of 5%. Infants with MAS are more likely to be delivered by Caesarean section due to fetal compromise. There is no evidence to suggest that MAS would be prevented if infants with meconium-stained liquor were delivered immediately, as the exact timing of the aspiration is not known.[5]

Cerebral palsy and intrapartum events

Epidemiological data suggest that only 10% of cases of cerebral palsy have a potential intrapartum cause.[4,14] For a diagnosis of cerebral palsy to be made as a result of intrapartum hypoxia certain criteria have to be met: evidence of metabolic acidosis, moderate to severe neonatal encephalopathy and the presence of either the spastic quadriplegic or dyskinetic type of the condition.

REFERENCES

1. K. B. Nelson, What proportion of cerebral palsy is related to birth asphyxia? *J. Pediatr.*, **112**:4 (1988), 572–4.

2. A. M. Vintzileos, D. J. Nochimson, E. R. Guzman *et al.*, Intrapartum electronic fetal heart rate monitoring versus intermittent auscultation: a meta-analysis. *Obstet. Gynecol.*, **85**:1 (1995), 149–55.

3. S. Thacker and D. Stroup, Continuous electronic heart rate monitoring versus intermittent auscultation for assessment during labour. *Cochrane Database Syst. Rev.*, 1999. Issue no. 3.

4. H. D. Modanlou and Y. Murata, Sinusoidal heart rate pattern: reappraisal of its definition and clinical significance. *J. Obstet. Gynaecol. Res.*, **30**:3 (2004), 169–80.

5. Clinical Effectiveness Support Unit of the Royal College of Obstetricians and Gynaecologists. *The Use and Interpretation of Cardiotocography in Intrapartum Fetal Surveillance – Evidence-based Clinical Guideline 8.* (London: RCOG Press, 2001).

6. ACOG technical bulletin, Fetal heart rate patterns: monitoring, interpretation, and management. Number 207 – July 1995 (replaces No. 132, September 1989). *Int. J. Gynaecol. Obstet.*, **51**:1 (1995), 65–74.

7. A. Elimian, R. Figueroa and N. Tejani, Intrapartum assessment of fetal well-being: a comparison of scalp stimulation with scalp blood pH sampling. *Obstet. Gynecol.*, **89**: 3 (1997), 373–6.

8. N. Lazebnik, M. R. Neuman, A. Lysikiewicz, L. R. Dierker and L. I. Mann, Response of fetal heart rate to scalp stimulation related to fetal acid–base status. *Am. J. Perinatol.*, **9**:4 (1992), 228–32.

9. J. A. Spencer, Predictive value of a fetal heart rate acceleration at the time of fetal blood sampling in labour. *J. Perinat. Med.*, **19**:3 (1991), 207–15.

10. R. Mistry and J. Neilson, Fetal electrocardiogram plus heart rate recording for fetal monitoring during labour. *Cochrane Database Syst. Rev.*, **2** (1999), CD000116.

11. B. K. Strachan, W. J. van Wijngaarden, D. Sahota, A. Chong and D. K. James, Cardiotocography only versus cardiotocography plus PR-interval analysis in intra-partum surveillance: a randomised, multicentre trial. FECG Study Group. *Lancet*, **355**:9202 (2000), 456–9.

12. N. A. Maclachlan, J. A. Spencer, K. Harding and S. Arulkumaran, Fetal acidaemia, the cardiotocograph and the T/QRS ratio of the fetal ECG in labour. *Br. J. Obstet. Gynaecol.*, **99**:1 (1992), 26–31.

13. G. A. Dildy, J. A. Thorp, J. D. Yeast and S. L. Clark, The relationship between oxygen saturation and pH in umbilical blood: implications for intrapartum fetal oxygen saturation monitoring. *Am. J. Obstet. Gynecol.*, **175**:3 Pt 1 (1996), 682–7.

14. *Confidential Enquiry into Stillbirths and Deaths in Infancy.* Seventh Annual Report. 1st January to 31st December 1998. (London: Maternal and Child Health Consortium, 2000).

FURTHER READING

S. M. Gauge and C. Henderson, *CTG Made Easy* 3rd edn (Edinburgh: Churchill Livingstone, 2005).

D. K. James, P. J. Steer, C. P. Weiner and B. Gonis, *High Risk Pregnancy: Management Options*, 3rd Edn (Edinburgh: Saunders, 2006).

L. H. Kean, P. N. Baker and D. I. Edelstone, *Best Practice in Labour Ward Management* (Philadelphia: Saunders, 2000).

T. Mitchell, *CTGs: Guidance for Interpretation: the Crimson File: a Selection of Cases Compiled During a Confidential Enquiry* (Solihull: West Midlands Perinatal Audit, 1995).

Pre-eclampsia and hypertensive disorders of pregnancy

Egidio da Silva and Wilson Chimbira

Introduction

Pre-eclampsia is a multi-system disorder, which primarily affects the cardiovascular system, leading to dysfunction of liver, lungs, kidney and brain. Pre-eclampsia is unpredictable in presentation and progression. At present, there is no curative treatment for pre-eclampsia and the ultimate management is the delivery of the fetus and placenta. Pre-eclampsia can present at any time after the 20th week of gestation, and is an important cause of iatrogenic prematurity, with the associated perinatal morbidity and mortality. In cases of extreme prematurity, pregnancy is prolonged until maternal health is at risk. Success in the management of pre-eclampsia is dependent at least in part on a multidisciplinary approach by the midwifery, obstetric, anaesthetic, intensive care and neonatal teams.

In the UK, pre-eclampsia has an incidence of between 3% and 5%, with severe pre-eclampsia complicating 0.5% of pregnancies.[1,2] Eclampsia affects only 0.05% of pregnancies in the UK.[2] It is estimated that 1 in 6 stillbirths and 14% of maternal mortality are due to pre-eclampsia and hypertensive disorders of pregnancy.[3]

Aetiology and pathogenesis

Pre-eclampsia is related to placental pathology, probably arising from decreased trophoblast invasion in the first trimester. This reduction in invasion fails to convert the convoluted spiral arteries to high-flow, low-resistance vessels that feed the placenta, thus decreasing placental blood flow, which may result in placental hypoxia and oxidative stress. It is hypothesised that the damaged placenta releases active factor(s) into the maternal circulation that results in endothelial damage and vasoconstriction within the maternal vasculature (Figure 7.1).[4] The presence of these active factors within the maternal circulation accounts for the multi-system nature of pre-eclampsia. Ultimately, delivery of the placenta, the proposed origin of these factors, terminates the clinical disorder.

Fetal complications of pre-eclampsia also result from placental dysfunction, and may be acute or chronic. Acute insults such as placental abruption may occur secondary to maternal hypertension. The presentation of chronic pathology depends on the duration and severity of the changes to the placenta, but may include intra-uterine growth restriction (IUGR), which may ultimately lead to intra-uterine fetal death (IUFD).

Obstetrics for Anaesthetists, ed. Alexander Heazell and John Clift. Published by Cambridge University Press © Cambridge University Press 2008

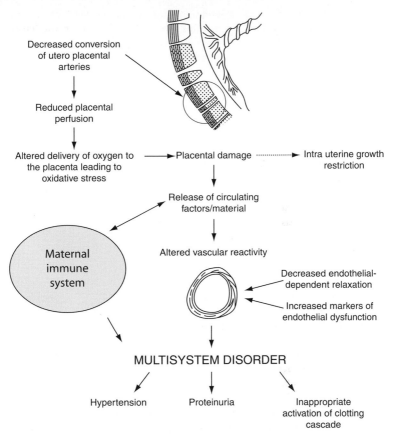

Figure 7.1 Proposed pathophysiology of pre-eclampsia, highlighting the roles of the placenta and the maternal immune system in the development of a multi-system disorder.

Definitions

Pre-existing hypertension is defined as a blood pressure >140/90 mmHg on 2 occasions 4 hours apart *before* 20 weeks gestation.

Pregnancy-induced hypertension (*PIH*) is defined as a blood pressure >140/90 mmHg on 2 occasions 4 hours apart *after* 20 weeks gestation.

Pre-eclampsia is defined as a blood pressure ≥140/90 mmHg, the development of hypertension with proteinuria greater than 0.3 g/24 hr or + + on urine dipstick testing after 20 weeks gestation.[5]

Superimposed pre-eclampsia describes the presence of new-onset proteinuria greater than 0.3 g/24 hr or + + on urine dipstick testing in a patient with pre-existing hypertension after 20 weeks gestation.

Eclampsia is the occurrence of fits, convulsions or coma without the presence of an underlying reason after 20 weeks of pregnancy. Eclampsia may occur prior to the onset of symptoms and signs of pre-eclampsia.

Diagnostic criteria

Pre-eclampsia[5]

Hypertension

- Blood pressure >140/90 mmHg on 2 or more consecutive occasions >4 hours apart
- Diastolic blood pressure >110 mmHg on one occasion

    Proteinuria

- >300 mg of protein in a 24-hour urine collection

    or

- 2 + or greater on a urinalysis strip

Severe pre-eclampsia

Severe hypertension

- Systolic blood pressure >160 mmHg

    or

- Diastolic blood pressure >110 mmHg on 2 occasions at least 6 hours apart during bed rest

AND

Proteinuria

Pre-eclampsia may also be classified as severe if there are symptoms or signs of end-organ involvement including:

- Central nervous system – severe headache, visual disturbances, clonus, hyper-reflexia, papilloedema
- Renal – decreased urine output
- Liver – epigastric pain, right upper quadrant pain, vomiting

    The presence of oedema is *not* a diagnostic criteria for pre-eclampsia. Ninety percent of patients in the third trimester will have pedal oedema.

Risk factors

Pre-existing:[1]

- Family history of pre-eclampsia (mother or sister)
- Increased maternal age (>40)

- Low socioeconomic status
- Maternal obesity
- Pre-existing hypertension
- Diabetes mellitus
- Autoimmune diseases e.g. SLE
- Inherited thrombophilias e.g. Factor V Leiden
- Renal disease
- Previous history of pre-eclampsia

Pregnancy-related factors:

- Primigravida
- First pregnancy with new partner
- Pregnancies conceived with assisted reproductive technologies especially if semen donor/egg donation
- Multiple pregnancy (twins/triplets)

Assessment of patients with hypertension and pre-eclampsia

An accurate clinical assessment of patients with hypertension and/or pre-eclampsia is essential as the clinical course, and subsequent management, is different for women with pregnancy-induced hypertension, pre-eclampsia and severe pre-eclampsia. Due to the multi-system nature of these disorders a thorough examination should be carried out.

Central nervous system

History
- Headache
- Visual disturbances
- General malaise
- Rarely, focal neurological symptoms e.g. limb weakness

Examination
- Hyper-reflexia
- Clonus
- Papilloedema
- Conjunctival haemorrhage
- Focal neurological deficit

Clinical features may be directly/indirectly caused by the following:
- Intense vasospasm of intracranial blood vessels
- Microvascular spasm in the retina

- Electrolyte imbalance
- Dramatic rise in blood pressure
- Impaired coagulation

A combination of these elements may lead to cerebrovascular accident.

Cardiovascular system

History
- Palpitations
- Shortness of breath
- Oedema – not specific for pre-eclampsia but may be sudden onset/upper body or face

Examination
- Raised blood pressure
- Low volume pulse/cool peripheries
- Tachycardia
- Poor capillary return

Clinical features may be directly/indirectly caused by the following:
- Decreased plasma protein
- Increased capillary fragility and permeability
- Decreased circulating volume and widespread vasoconstriction
- Increased systemic vascular resistance
- Left ventricular failure in the most severe cases

Respiratory system

History
- Facial oedema
- Hoarse voice
- Shortness of breath

Examination
- Stridor and tachypnoea
- Decreased air entry
- Fine inspiratory crepitations in lung bases

Clinical features may be directly/indirectly caused by the following:
- Extensive oedema, which may include laryngeal oedema
- Pulmonary oedema
- Rarely, adult respiratory distress syndrome may develop

Gastrointestinal system

History
- Nausea and vomiting
- Epigastric or right upper quadrant pain
- General malaise

Examination
- Severe upper abdominal tenderness

Investigations
- Liver function tests (LFTs) may identify elevated transaminase levels and decreased albumin
- Alkaline phosphatase levels are elevated in pregnancy due to placental alkaline phosphatase

Clinical features may be directly/indirectly caused by the following:
- Liver dysfunction resulting from periportal necrosis
- Stretching of the liver capsule or rarely by subcapsular liver haemorrhage (constant lower abdominal pain may be indicative of placental abruption)

Renal system

History
- Decreased urine output
- Shortness of breath
- Oedema – not specific for pre-eclampsia but may be sudden onset/upper body or face

Examination
- Widespread oedema

Investigation
- Renal function tests (U&Es), urea and creatinine normally lower in pregnancy than non-pregnant levels. May be elevated in pre-eclampsia.
- Serum uric acid; plasma uric acid concentrations $>360\,\mu$mol/l are associated with pre-eclampsia, and are thought to reflect renal impairment.[6]
- Urinanalysis/24-hour urine collection.

Clinical features may be directly/indirectly caused by the following:
- Increased endothelial permeability, which leads to proteinuria.

- Reversible glomerular endothelial lesion causing temporary compromise of renal function. If complicated by hypovolaemia, acute tubular necrosis may result.
- Reduced renal blood flow and glomerular filtration rate in most patients

In more severe cases acute renal failure may occur, although there are few reports.

Assessment of haematological and clotting parameters

History
- Spontaneous bleeding e.g. haematuria, antepartum haemorrhage
- Moderately increased risk of thromboembolism

Examination
- Spontaneous bleeding from injection sites or mucous membranes
- Signs of anaemia (pale mucous membranes, shortness of breath)
- Signs of thromboembolism/deep vein thrombosis (DVT)

Investigations
- Full blood count (FBC) (haemoglobin, platelets)
- Clotting studies (PT, APTT)

Clinical features may be directly/indirectly caused by the following:
- Endothelial activation/inappropriate consuming clotting factors and platelets in small vessels, allowing bleeding from other sites.
- Severe variant of pre-eclampsia termed HELLP syndrome (**h**aemolysis, **e**levated **l**iver enzymes, **l**ow **p**latelets)

Assessment of fetus

History
- Antepartum haemorrhage
- Lower abdominal pain
- Reduced fetal movements

Examination
- Incongruence between gestational age and fundal height suggesting a small-for-gestational-age/IUGR fetus.
- Lower abdominal tenderness, hard tender uterus

Investigations
- Auscultation of fetal heart/cardiotocography (depending on gestational age)
- Ultrasound scan

Clinical features may be directly/indirectly caused by the following:
- Placental insufficiency
- Placental abruption

Management of pre-eclampsia and pregnancy-induced hypertension

The main aims of management are:
- To ensure survival of the mother with minimal morbidity
- To ensure that the fetus is delivered as close to term as possible

Important aspects in the management of pre-eclampsia are:
- Blood pressure control
- Prevention of eclamptic fits
- Fluid balance
- Delivery of the fetus
- Effective postpartum care
- Management of complications e.g. eclampsia/HELLP syndrome

Pregnancy-induced hypertension

Women with asymptomatic pregnancy-induced hypertension >140/90 and < 160/110 mmHg can be successfully assessed as outpatients via a day assessment unit, allowing the clinician to commence and monitor the effect of anti-hypertensive medication.[7] However, over 40% of patients will go on to develop pre-eclampsia.[8] Therefore, monitoring blood pressure, proteinuria, renal, liver and haematological function is essential. Patients with a blood pressure >160/100 mmHg require immediate assessment by an obstetrician, and are likely to require admission to hospital for bed rest, anti-hypertensive medication and regular monitoring of blood pressure (at least every 4 hours).[7]

Pre-eclampsia

Due to the unpredictable nature of the disease, women with pre-eclampsia require close surveillance to allow intervention prior to deterioration of maternal or fetal condition. Patients with blood pressure >160/100 mmHg with proteinuria require immediate admission to hospital; women with blood pressure >140/90 mmHg, proteinuria and symptoms of pre-eclampsia should also be admitted for observation.

Blood pressure control

Treatment of pre-existing hypertension does not improve the fetal outcome, but reduces the incidence of severe hypertension. In addition, there is some evidence to suggest that pregnancy can be prolonged by expectant management of pre-eclampsia, with blood pressure control and appropriate investigations. However, the control of blood pressure does not prevent deterioration of pre-eclampsia or the perinatal morbidity. The use of expectant management will depend upon the gestation of the patient; a patient presenting at 26 weeks' gestation should receive expectant management, whereas a patient at 38 weeks has achieved fetal maturity, and expectant management will achieve little or no benefit. Blood pressure control in pregnancy differs from that outside pregnancy in that the goal of treatment is not to achieve "normal" values, but to reduce the risk of maternal cerebrovascular damage.

When to treat:

- Treatment should be commenced if blood pressure >160/100 mmHg[9]
- Treatment should be considered at lower blood pressures if there are other markers of severe disease (+++ proteinuria or maternal symptoms)[9]
- Pre-existing hypertension, early in pregnancy

How to treat:

- Acute reduction in blood pressure can be achieved using labetalol (oral or intravenous), nifedipine (orally) or hydralazine (intravenously). Brief information is shown in Table 7.1 (See Chapter 13 for further information on therapeutic agents)
- Oral methyldopa can be used for longer-term management especially for pre-existing hypertension
- Nifedipine should *not* be given sublingually – potentially causes a large reduction in utero placental blood flow precipitating fetal distress[10]

> During labour, epidural analgesia is effective in reducing blood pressure.

Fluid balance

Maintenance of fluid balance is essential in the management of severe pre-eclampsia, to prevent iatrogenic pulmonary oedema due to fluid overload. The likelihood of pulmonary oedema complicating pre-eclampsia is increased by vasoconstriction, decreased circulating volume (up to 40% in severe cases), low oncotic pressure and poor left ventricular function. Close monitoring of fluid balance facilitates early identification of renal impairment.

- Patients with severe pre-eclampsia should be catheterised and a strict chart of fluid balance should be kept.[9]
- Fluid restrict using crystalloid/clear fluids at 1 ml/kg/hr or 2 l/24 hours.[9]
- Oliguria is common in pre-eclamptic patients, although acute renal failure is rare.
- Urine output should remain >0.5 ml/kg/hr, although no evidence that maintaining a specific urine output prevents acute renal failure.
- If severely oliguric, give 500 ml bolus of crystalloid; if no improvement in urine output, consider central venous pressure (CVP) monitoring. The use of CVP is controversial and there is poor correlation between CVP and left-sided cardiac filling pressures.

Table 7.1 Commonly used antihypertensive agents indicating their time of use

Drug	Use	Important notes	Drug dose
Methyldopa	A, P	Slow onset of action, normally used to control pre-existing hypertension or mild PIH. Haemolysis may occur	0.5–3 g/24 hours in 3 divided doses
Nifedipine	A, I, P	Rapid onset. Sublingual form should not be given. Side effects include headache and oedema	10 mg of oral form given (rapid onset) followed by 10–20 mg of modified release form upto 8 hourly
Hydralazine	A, I, P	Rapid onset of action. Side effects of overdose similar to symptoms of severe pre-eclampsia e.g. headache, tremors	Intravenous loading dose 10–20 mg administered over 10–20 minutes, followed by infusion 1–5 mg/hr
Labetalol	A, I, P	Alpha- and beta-blocker, rapid onset of action. Should be avoided in asthmatics	200 mg orally, if ineffective loading dose 50 mg followed by infusion of 20–160 mg/hr

A = Antepartum, I = Intrapartum, P = Postpartum.

- Platelets, blood or other blood products may be used as required (they will have a similar effect to colloids in their effect on the cardiovascular system).
- Urea and electrolytes should be monitored regularly.
- Diuretics are ineffective hypotensive agents in pregnancy, and are likely to deplete fluid in the intravascular space and should be avoided unless there is evidence of pulmonary oedema.

If there are signs of poor or worsening renal function advice should be sought from intensive care and nephrology physicians.

Hypotension may occur due to anti-hypertensive agents, regional anaesthesia and analgesia.

During regional anaesthesia for operative delivery:
- Pre-loading with fluid should be minimised due to risks of pulmonary oedema.
- Hypotension should be treated with careful administration of IV fluids and vasopressors.
- Blood loss during surgery should be replaced with fluids.
- If blood loss occurs invasive monitoring should be instituted earlier than in non-pre-eclamptic patients, as estimation of fluid balance is more difficult.

Table 7.2 Clinical signs of magnesium toxicity and related plasma magnesium concentrations

	Plasma levels (mmol/l)
Therapeutic levels	2.0–4.0
ECG changes (wide QRS, prolonged PR)	3.0–5.0
Loss of deep tendon reflexes	> 5.0
Heart block, CNS and respiratory depression	> 7.5
Cardiac arrest	> 12

Prevention and treatment of eclamptic seizures

Magnesium sulphate is the agent of choice for both prevention and treatment of eclamptic fits.

Prevention

- Magnesium sulphate should be considered for women who have severe pre-eclampsia (see Diagnostic criteria), as it reduces the incidence of seizures by 58% and decreases maternal mortality.[11,12]
- Magnesium should be continued for 24 hours post delivery or 24 hours after the last seizure/neurological signs whichever is the latter.
- Regular assessments of urine output, maternal reflexes, respiratory rate and oxygen saturations should be made to identify signs of magnesium toxicity (see Table 7.2).
- There is no need to monitor plasma magnesium levels routinely.
- Magnesium levels should be monitored if the urine output is < 100 ml/4hours (magnesium is excreted renally).
- Symptoms of magnesium toxicity are weakness, nausea, double vision, slurred speech, drowsiness and flushing sensations. Unfortunately, these may be confused with central nervous system symptoms of eclampsia.
- Magnesium should be stopped if the deep tendon reflexes are absent, until they return, and if there is a reduction in respiratory rate.
- If severe respiratory depression or respiratory arrest calcium gluconate 1 g (10 ml) should be given IV over 10 minutes. Magnesium levels should be checked and infusions stopped if toxicity is thought to be a possibility.

Magnesium regime (example):
- Loading dose, 4 g (made up to 40 ml infused at 240 ml/hr)
- Maintenance, 1–2 g/hr (5 g made up to 50 ml infused at 10–20 ml/hr)

Magnesium:
- Prolongs the action of non-depolarizing muscle relaxants
- Reduces suxamethonium fasciculations

  Nerve stimulators should be used when patients treated with magnesium are having a general anaesthetic.

Eclampsia

- Eclamptic fits may present in the antepartum (30%), intrapartum (30%) and postpartum (40%) periods
- Eclampsia may precede signs and symptoms of pre-eclampsia, and severity of hypertension does not correlate with the incidence of fits
- Signs and symptoms of impending eclampsia include hyper-reflexia, visual disturbances, headache and abdominal pain
- Eclamptic seizures are generalised and self-limiting
- 1–2% of women will have persistent neurological damage following an eclamptic fit

Treatment

- Initial treatment follows the basic principles **A**irway, **B**reathing and **C**irculation.
- IV access should be obtained.
- 4 g magnesium sulphate is used to control the seizure (see treatment regime).
- For recurrent seizures a further 2 g bolus of magnesium is given and the maintenance increased to 20 ml/hr (2 g/hr).
- It should also be ascertained that the patient has not aspirated during an unwitnessed convulsion – chest X-ray may be indicated.
- If antepartum, a fit is often accompanied by a fetal bradycardia (due to maternal hypoxia) – *the primary concern is the wellbeing of the mother*. Adequate resuscitation and stabilisation of maternal condition will resuscitate the fetus.

Recurrent and resistant fits:
- Magnesium (2 g bolus)
- Single dose of IV diazepam
- Rarely, thiopentone, intubation and Critical Care transfer may be indicated

Observations and investigations for severe pre-eclampsia/eclampsia

- Patients should be managed in a 1:1 environment (many delivery suites have a high-dependency area)
- Continuous monitoring SaO_2 and pulse
- Non-invasive blood pressure every 15 minutes
- Accurate hourly fluid input and output (catheterise)
- FBC, U&E, LFT and clotting studies every 12–24 hours

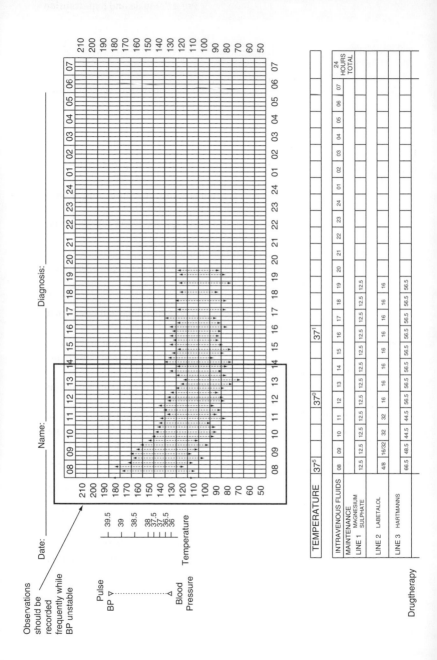

Observations should be recorded frequently while BP unstable

Date: _____   Name: _____   Diagnosis: _____

Pulse
BP ▽ ⋯⋯⋯⋯⋯⋯⋯ △ Blood Pressure

Temperature

TEMPERATURE	37.5			37.0				37.1					37.0		

	08	09	10	11	12	13	14	15	16	17	18	19	20	21	22	23	24	01	02	03	04	05	06	07
INTRAVENOUS FLUIDS																								
MAINTENANCE LINE 1 MAGNESIUM SULPHATE	12.5	12.5	12.5	12.5	12.5	12.5	12.5	12.5	12.5	12.5	12.5	12.5												
LINE 2 LABETALOL	4/8	16/32	32	32	16	16	16	16	16	16	16	16												
LINE 3 HARTMANNS	66.5	48.5	44.5	44.5	56.5	56.5	56.5	56.5	56.5	56.5	56.5	56.5												

	07	06	05	04	03	02	01	24	23	22	21	20	07	06	05	04	03	02	01	24 HOURS TOTAL

Drugtherapy

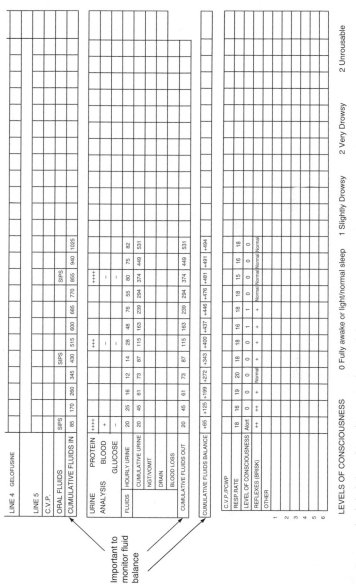

Figure 7.2 Example of a high dependency chart to record maternal observations in patients with severe pre-eclampsia or eclampsia, enabling the recording of blood pressure, fluid balance, and medication on a single record.

LEVELS OF CONSCIOUSNESS   0 Fully awake or light/normal sleep   1 Slightly Drowsy   2 Very Drowsy   2 Unrousable

- Intra-arterial blood pressure and CVP/Pulmonary capillary wedge pressure monitoring for more severe cases especially if there is doubt re fluid balance[13]
- The use of a high-dependency chart provides a valuable overview of the patient's condition Figure 7.2

Delivery following severe pre-eclampsia or eclampsia

Once the maternal condition is stabilised, the next priority is delivery of the baby. The timing, place and mode of delivery will depend on the gestation of the infant, the presence of neonatal facilities (if required) and the probability of delivery. Patients with severe pre-eclampsia or eclampsia often labour and deliver rapidly, and if suitable for induction of labour, this may be the preferred option, as Caesarean section will lead to greater blood loss and increased risk of venous thromboembolism. However, if there is evidence of fetal distress, prematurity or other contraindications to induction of labour, delivery will be achieved by Caesarean section.

Maternal diastolic blood pressure should be stabilised below of 100 mmHg prior to delivery by Caesarean section.

Irrespective of the mode of delivery, regional anaesthesia has the benefit of further reducing maternal blood pressure due to venous pooling of blood; both spinal and epidural anaesthesia are considered safe providing platelets are $>80 \times 10^{12}$/l and there is no evidence of coagulopathy. Furthermore, if available continuous low-dose local anaesthetic infusions are probably more efficient in maintaining a steady state of placental blood flow and blood pressure levels than bolus dose methods.

Hypotension occurring during Caesarean section or following regional anaesthesia is treated by careful fluid resuscitation (crystalloid, colloid or blood and blood products but beware of causing pulmonary oedema). Vasopressors, such as phenylephrine, ephedrine or metaraminol, should be given very carefully and in much smaller doses than are normally used due to the exaggerated vasoconstrictor response in pre-eclampsia/pregnancy-induced hypertension.

Epidural analgesia
- Establish epidural analgesia early in labour.
- If platelets $>100 \times 10^9$/l regional anaesthesia may be performed without checking clotting studies.
- Regional anaesthesia is contraindicated if platelets $< 80 \times 10^9$/l.
- If platelet count is between 80 and 100×10^9/l the clotting studies should be checked and the INR < 1.5 is considered safe.
- Enables good blood pressure control, a controlled reduction in blood pressure and can be used to anaesthetise for Caesarean section.
- Improves placental perfusion due to peripheral vasodilatation.
- Use low doses of local anaesthetic and opiates.

> **Intubation in patients with pre-eclampsia/eclampsia**
>
> - Airway management may be difficult due to oedema of the face, mouth, neck and oropharynx. Also potentially difficult to secure an urgent surgical airway.
> - Increased risk of bleeding – worsens the success rate for fibreoptic intubation due to nasopharyngeal oedema as well as bleeding risk.
> - Increased risk of intracerebral bleed due to severe hypertension.
> - Care must be taken to decrease the pressor response to intubation.
> - Alfentanil (10 μg/kg), labetalol (10–20 mg) and magnesium (40 mg/kg) may be used prior to induction, to obtund the response to intubation.
> - Care with the pressor response should also be taken on extubation.
> - Post-operative airway obstruction may occur as a result of laryngeal oedema.

Following delivery, the third stage of labour should be managed using 5 units oxytocin given IM or IV to prevent postpartum haemorrhage.[9] Syntometrine or ergometrine should be avoided as these agents will further increase blood pressure.

Postpartum management

Women with severe pre-eclampsia and eclampsia require close monitoring after delivery. Normally, blood pressure and urine output return to normal in the 24 hours postpartum.

- If blood pressure is not stable it should be measured every 15 minutes; when blood pressure has stabilised at safe levels frequency of blood pressure monitoring can be decreased.
- Control of fluid balance – urine output should be monitored.
- Fluid intake can be increased when urine output increases.
- Anti-hypertensive medication should be titrated to blood pressure, but should not be stopped abruptly – this will lead to rebound hypertension.
- Intravenous anti-hypertensive agents should be transferred to oral therapy if longer-term blood pressure control is required.
- Magnesium sulphate should be continued for 24 hours after delivery or for 24 hours after the last seizure whichever is longer.
- Patients with pre-eclampsia are considered to be at moderate risk of developing thromboembolism and it is recommended that they should receive low molecular weight heparin prophylaxis. However, this is contraindicated if there is a deficiency in platelets and/or clotting factors.

All women with pre-eclampsia or hypertension need careful review by an experienced clinician prior to discharge. Anti-hypertensive medication may need to be continued for up to 3 months. Persistent hypertension and proteinuria will require investigation by a renal physician.

Women with severe pre-eclampsia and eclampsia have an increased risk of hypertension, pre-eclampsia and eclampsia in subsequent pregnancies.

Management of HELLP syndrome

Haemolysis, elevated liver enzymes and low platelets describe the syndrome that is a consumptive coagulopathy. The haemolysis results in anaemia.

- Periportal haemorrhage and necrosis results in hepatic ischaemia leading to hepatic dysfunction.
- Serum haptoglobin concentrations may be used to detect haemolysis at an early stage. Peripheral blood film may detect red cell fragments.
- HELLP syndrome may precede hypertension or proteinuria, and is more common in multiparous women.
- HELLP syndrome can occur in the postpartum period in 20–25 % of cases.
- Should be ruled out in patients complaining of epigastric or right upper quadrant pain, headaches, malaise, blurring of vision, nausea, vomiting or presenting with haematuria (urinalysis unreliable in the presence of blood per vagina).
- HELLP has a high fetal mortality and maternal mortality is higher than other presentations of pre-eclampsia. If HELLP syndrome occurs antenatally, delivery is the ideal treatment.
- Active and immediate treatment of haematological abnormalities should be instituted and a haematologist should be involved at an early stage in the management of HELLP syndrome. Otherwise the management is the same as for severe pre-eclampsia.

REFERENCES

1. J. E. Myers and J. Brockelsby, The epidemiology of pre-eclampsia. In P. N. Baker and J. C. P. Kingdom eds., *Pre-eclampsia: Current Perspectives on Management* (London: Parthenon, 2004), pp. 25–39.
2. D. J. Tuffnell, D. Jankowicz, S. W. Lindow *et al.*, Outcomes of severe pre-eclampsia/ eclampsia in Yorkshire 1999–2003. *Br. J. Obstet. Gynaecol.*, **112**:7 (2005), 875–80.
3. Confidential Enquiry into Maternal and Child Health, *Why Mothers Die* 2000–2002 – The Sixth Report of the Confidential Enquiries into Maternal Deaths in the United Kingdom (London: RCOG Press, 2004).
4. M. C. Mushambi, A. W. Halligan and K. Williamson, Recent developments in the pathophysiology and management of pre-eclampsia. *Br. J. Anaesth.*, **76** (1996), 133–48.
5. D. A. Davey and I. MacGillivray, The classification and definition of the hypertensive disorders of pregnancy. *Am. J. Obstet. Gynecol.*, **158**:4 (1988), 892–8.
6. L. K. Wagner, Diagnosis and management of pre-eclampsia. *Am. Fam. Physician* **70**:12 (2004), 2317–24.

7. F. Milne, C. Redman, J. Walker *et al.*, The pre-eclampsia community guideline (PRECOG): how to screen for and detect onset of pre-eclampsia in the community. *BMJ*, **330**:7491 (2005), 576–80.

8. J. R. Barton, J. M. O'Brien, N. K. Bergauer, D. L. Jacques and B. M. Sibai, Mild gestational hypertension remote from term: progression and outcome. *Am. J. Obstet. Gynecol.*, **184**:5 (2001), 979–83.

9. Royal College of Obstetricians and Gynaecologists. *The Management of Severe Pre-eclampsia/Eclampsia.* Guideline 10(A) (London: RCOG Press, 2006).

10. L. Impey, Severe hypotension and fetal distress following sublingual administration of nifedipine to a patient with severe pregnancy induced hypertension at 33 weeks. *Br. J. Obstet. Gynaecol.*, **100** (1993), 959–61.

11. L. Duley, A. M. Gulmezoglu and D. J. Henderson-Smart, Magnesium sulphate and other anticonvulsants for women with pre-eclampsia. *Cochrane Database Syst. Rev.*, **3** (2006), CD000025.

12. D. Altman, G. Carroli, L. Duley *et al.*, Do women with pre-eclampsia, and their babies, benefit from magnesium sulphate? The Magpie Trial: a randomised placebo-controlled trial. *Lancet*, **359**:9321 (2002), 1877–90.

13. S. L. Clark, J. S. Greenspoon and D. Aldahl, Severe pre-eclampsia with persistent oliguria: management of hemodynamic subsets. *Am. J. Obstet. Gynecol.*, **154** (1986), 490–4.

FURTHER READING

M. F. M. James, Magnesium in obstetric anesthesia. *Int. J. Obstet. Anesth.*, **7**(1998), 115–23.

Practice Guidelines for Obstetrical Anesthesia. *Anesthesiology*, **90** (1999), 600–11.

J. J. Walker, Severe pre-eclampsia and eclampsia. *Best Pract. Res. Clin. Obstet. Gynaecol.*, **14** (2000), 57–71.

Operative obstetrics

Jo Gillham

Introduction

Deviation from a 'normal vaginal delivery' is a frequent event in modern day obstetrics, and may be for fetal and/or maternal reasons. Instrumental delivery can be achieved through the use of many types of vacuum extractor and with different makes of forceps. The rate of instrumental delivery rates is remaining stable at approximately 10–15%.[1] Vaginal delivery may not be achievable or indeed not attempted and this will necessitate delivery via the abdominal route 'Caesarean section'. The incidence of delivery by Caesarean section is approximately 20% and rising.[1]

Caesarean section

Indications for Caesarean section

The indications for the Caesarean section are organised into four categories, depending on how quickly the operation needs to be performed.[2]

1 – Immediate threat to life of women or fetus
   Examples include: prolonged fetal bradycardia, umbilical cord prolapse, uterine rupture, fetal scalp pH < 7.2, placental abruption

2 – Maternal or fetal compromise but not immediately life-threatening
   Examples include: failure to progress in labour, failed induction of labour

3 – No maternal or fetal compromise but needs early delivery
   Examples include: patient booked for planned Caesarean section presenting with rupture of membranes

4 – Delivery times to suit woman or staff[2]
   Examples include: elective Caesarean section for breech presentation, twins or previous Caesarean section

> The decision to delivery interval for a category 1 Caesarean section should be less than 30 minutes.

> There is much controversy surrounding the use of general and regional anaesthesia for a category 1 Caesarean section. Each case must be assessed individually. In principle, the considerations are that the decision to delivery time should be less than 30 minutes (sometimes much less) and mother's safety is paramount.

Obstetrics for Anaesthetists, ed. Alexander Heazell and John Clift. Published by Cambridge University Press. © Cambridge University Press 2008

The time interval for a category 2 Caesarean section is less clear and there is little evidence to guide practice. The National Caesarean Section Sentinel Audit showed that there were no harmful consequences provided delivery occurred within 75 minutes.[1]

> Unless contraindicated, regional anaesthesia is the anaesthetic of choice for category 2, 3 and 4 Caesarean sections.

Preparation for Caesarean section

Prior to Caesarean section all women should:
- Give valid informed consent
- Have haemoglobin (Hb) checked to assess for anaemia
- If there is increased risk of bleeding take blood for grouping and saving of serum or cross-matching if appropriate
- Have risk of thrombosis assessed and appropriate intervention prescribed including graduated compression stockings
- Have bladder catheterised

> There is an increased risk of > 1000 ml blood loss at Caesarean section in the following conditions:
> - Antepartum haemorrhage (particularly placenta praevia or massive placental abruption)
> - Uterine rupture
> - > 2 previous Caesarean sections
>
> This should be anticipated – patients should have $2 \times$ large-bore cannulae, fluid can be given through a warming device and blood cross-matched ready for use

> ### Indications for cross-matching blood
> - Placenta praevia
> - Bleeding diathesis
> - Two or more previous Caesarean sections
> - Multiple pregnancy
> - Polyhydramnios
> - Hb < 10 g/dl
> - Anticipated laboratory difficulties in cross-matching/obtaining blood

Procedure for lower segment Caesarean section

The majority of deliveries are achieved through a low transverse abdominal skin incision and a transverse incision through the lower segment of the uterus (Figure 8.1). This achieves better cosmetic appearance and wound healing on

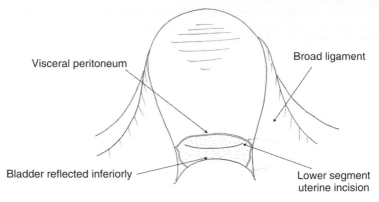

Figure 8.1 Site of uterine incision in lower segment Caesarean section.

the abdominal skin.[1] This requires decreased analgesic requirements and has less respiratory compromise in the post-operative period. A single transverse incision in the lower uterine segment allows an attempt at a vaginal delivery in the next pregnancy providing there are no other contraindications. The patients are counselled that there is an approximate risk of 1 in 200 of scar dehiscence during the labour. However, after 2 lower segment incisions have been performed on a uterus, patients are counselled that attempting a delivery via the vaginal route is unwise, due to the substantial risk in scar dehiscence/uterine rupture. Abdominal entry becomes progressively more difficult and potentially more time consuming with previous abdominal surgery.

Practical surgical steps during a Caesarean section

- The skin is opened with a scalpel. If there is an old scar present in an appropriate position, a repeat incision through that scar will be performed, and the option to excise the old scar is available.
- The incision of choice should then be the Cohen incision, transverse and 3 cm above the symphysis pubis.[2] A vertical skin incision may be required in extreme obesity or if other abdominal pathology is suspected or known to be present, but is not routinely required to do a classical Caesarean section.
- The subcutaneous tissues are dissected in the midline to the rectus sheath with sharp dissection. The remainder of the sheath can be exposed by sharp or blunt dissection.
- The rectus sheath is incised transversely in the middle 2 cm with the scalpel and the incision extended with the curved Mayo scissors.

- The fascial sheath is then separated from the underlying rectus muscle by sharp or blunt dissection – techniques being operator dependent and varying on the presence of scar tissue from previous operations.
- The rectus muscle is parted vertically and the abdominal peritoneum opened. With previous surgery, extra care must be taken to avoid damage to bladder or bowel.
- The uterus and bladder are then exposed. The utero-vesical peritoneum is then divided and the bladder reflected down to allow an incision to be made in the lower segment of the uterus. Previous scarring can make this peritoneal reflection sub-optimal, requiring a transverse incision slightly higher on the uterus but still in the anatomical lower segment.
- A transverse uterine incision is made with a scalpel in the upper layers, but final entry to the uterus should be bluntly achieved with a finger to minimise fetal lacerations during surgery and to reduce blood loss.[2] Delivery is then achieved.
- Occasionally delivery of the fetus will be more difficult than anticipated and the transverse incision will need to be extended sometimes into the upper segment of the uterus. These are the 'J' incision (an extension upwards from one angle of the transverse incision) or an 'inverted T' incision, where the original incision is extended upwards in the midline (Figure 8.2). These incisions are to be avoided unless necessary as they will lead to a contraindication for vaginal delivery in a subsequent pregnancy due to the risk of uterine rupture.

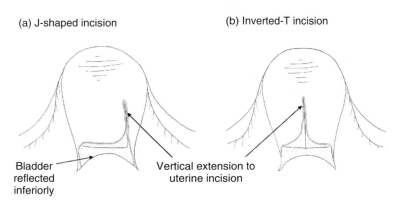

(a) J-shaped incision   (b) Inverted-T incision

Bladder reflected inferiorly

Vertical extension to uterine incision

Figure 8.2 Possible extensions to the uterine incision for lower segment Caesarean section showing either (a) a J-shaped extension connected to the lateral angle of the incision or (b) an inverted-T extension connected to the centre of the lower segment incision.

Uterine relaxation, to assist a difficult delivery, may be provided by:
- Sublingual or intravenous glyceryl trinitrate
- Increasing the concentration of the inspired volatile agent during general anaesthesia

- Once the fetal presenting part is at the uterine incision, fundal pressure is needed to achieve delivery.
- After delivery, an oxytocic (5 units IV oxytocin) and prophylactic antibiotics are administered (e.g. cephalosporin and metronidazole).
- The placenta is removed by controlled cord traction or if adherent manual removal may be required.
- Repair of the uterine incision can normally be achieved with the uterus *in situ*. However, if there have been extensions to the incision margins, it may be necessary to exteriorise the uterus to facilitate surgical repair.

Exteriorisation of the uterus increases pain and conversion of regional to general anaesthesia. It should not be done unless absolutely necessary.

- Green–Armitage forceps are placed around the uterine incision to improve visualisation of the incision angles and to reduce blood loss whilst suturing is commenced. Closure of the uterus in the UK is generally a double layer technique (unless in the context of a trial or if a clinical indication is present), with an absorbable suture such as vicryl.
- The parietal and abdominal peritoneum are not routinely sutured (this causes increased post-operative pain and adhesions).
- The paracolic gutters are cleaned with a swab on a stick to remove blood and amniotic fluid.
- The rectus sheath is closed with an absorbable suture such as vicryl.
- Routine closure of the subcutaneous tissues is not recommended, unless the patient has > 2 cm subcutaneous fat, as there is no evidence that this reduces wound infection.[1]
- Skin closure can be achieved with a subcuticular running suture (both absorbable and non-absorbable suture material), interrupted non-absorbable sutures (especially if the patient is at increased risk of a wound haematoma) or staples.
- Drains are not routinely used. However they can be placed in the pelvic cavity, above the rectus sheath or in the subcuticular space if the patient is felt to be at an increased risk of bleeding.
- It is routine to offer women delivered by Caesarean section thromboprophylaxis. This may be early mobilisation and graduated compression stockings in a low-risk patient having an uncomplicated elective Caesarean section, to low

molecular weight heparin for higher-risk patients and those having an emergency Caesarean section.[3] Most units have developed guidelines for the use of thromboprophylaxis as thromboembolism is still the leading cause of maternal death (see Chapter 10).[4]

The stages of Caesarean section likely to cause most discomfort to the patient are:
- Stretching of rectus sheath – as opposed to dissection
- Fundal pressure to deliver baby
- Exteriorisation of uterus
- Cleaning paracolic gutters

Classical Caesarean section

A classical Caesarean section is not dependent on the skin incision but on the uterine incision. If the uterine incision is made or extends into the upper segment of the uterus this is termed a 'classical'. The implication is that a vaginal delivery would be contraindicated in a subsequent pregnancy due to increased risk of uterine rupture compared to the incision in the lower uterine segment. There are few absolute indications for a classical Caesarean section. Certainly this incision is considered in situations such as: lower uterine segment containing anterior fibroids, premature delivery that may be too traumatic to the fetus through a transverse incision, avoidance of an anterior low-lying placenta.

The main differences in the procedure are:
- The bladder does not need to (cannot) be reflected.
- The uterine incision is performed in the midline of the uterus in the upper pole (Figure 8.3).

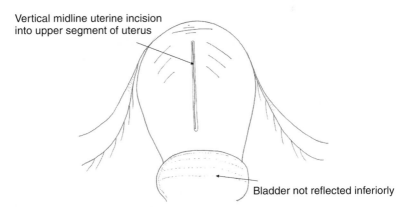

Vertical midline uterine incision into upper segment of uterus

Bladder not reflected inferiorly

Figure 8.3 Site of uterine incision in a classical Caesarean section, note that this does not necessarily need to be accompanied by a vertical skin incision.

- The uterine cavity cannot be entered bluntly due to the thickness of the upper segment. The initial uterine incision can be made with the knife and once the cavity is opened, can be extended with scissors/knife as necessary.
- The uterus is more likely to need to be exteriorised to facilitate suturing and a minimum of three layer closure is required thus increasing blood loss and operative time.
- If a vertical skin incision has been used, then mass closure of the abdominal wall should be employed with a slowly absorbable continuous suture as this will result in fewer incisional hernias and less wound dehiscence than layered closure.[2]

Classical Caesarean section:
- Increases post-operative pain (especially if vertical skin incision used)
- Increases operative time
- Increases blood loss compared to lower segment Caesarean section

---

Complications of Caesarean section including Caesarean hysterectomy

Although the incidence of Caesarean section is increasing it should not be forgotten that this is a major abdominal procedure and thus carries with it inherent risks.

Intra-operative complications

Urinary tract damage

Direct injury to the bladder can occur during entry into the abdomen (e.g. higher risk in previous abdominal surgery and after prolonged labours with caudally displaced oedematous bladders). Pre-operative catheterisation and careful technique should help prevent this. Damage to the ureters is uncommon as reflection of the bladder displaces them rostrally; however, abnormal anatomy, previous surgery and extensions of the uterine incision all increase the likelihood of damage. In most instances, a urologist will be required to complete the surgical repair and dictate necessary post-operative care and investigations.

Bowel damage

Bowel damage is rare at Caesarean section, but again is increased if there has been previous abdominal surgery. Repair is best conducted in conjunction with a general surgeon.

Haemorrhage

The average blood loss at a routine Caesarean section is 500 ml. A recent study has suggested that the transfusion incidence is in the region of 2–3%.[5] It found that marked increased risks were severe pre-operative anaemia and Caesarean section with a low-lying placenta.

Caesarean hysterectomy

The most common indication for Caesarean section hysterectomy is uncontrollable maternal haemorrhage. This may be secondary to uterine atony, due to extensions of the uterine incision during delivery, uterine rupture or secondary to a morbidly adherent placenta. For uterine atony as well as additional medical treatment (see Chapter 9 on Obstetric haemorrhage) surgical manipulation can be employed. B-lynch sutures can be tied around the uterus to attempt to compress the enlarged uterus. Ligation of the internal iliac arteries can be attempted to decrease the uterine blood supply. There is an increasing role for embolisation of the internal iliac arteries by an interventional radiologist. In antenatal high-risk cases there is the opportunity to place stents into the internal iliac arteries immediately pre-operative. If haemorrhage should occur, balloons in these stents can be inflated to decrease the blood supply to the uterus. This may be much more difficult to achieve in an emergency situation.

Obstetric haemorrhage is an emergency and extra personnel are needed with consultant anaesthetist and obstetrician being present and the haematologist and laboratory informed of the emergency and need for blood products. There is no clinical standard as to when a Caesarean hysterectomy is recommended. Most clinicians would accept that if the blood loss remains uncontrollable after 3 litres, careful consideration to this intervention is warranted.

Post-operative complications

Infection

Urine, wound and uterine infections are the commonest complications after a Caesarean section. The use of prophylactic antibiotics at Caesarean section has significantly reduced the incidence.

Venous thromboembolism

This has been mentioned previously. There were 30 deaths in the three years from 2000–2, making this still the leading cause of direct maternal mortality in the UK. Ten of these were after Caesarean section and eight women had additional risk factors other than pregnancy and operative delivery. The analysis of care was felt to be substandard in seven cases.[4]

Instrumental vaginal delivery

When an instrumental delivery is required it may be for fetal and/or maternal reasons. Fetal reasons include fetal malposition (occipito-transverse or posterior), and presumed fetal compromise.

Maternal reasons include maternal exhaustion and/or prolongation of the second stage of labour (if active second stage of labour 'pushing' is longer than 1 hour for a primigravida, or 45 minutes for a multipara), maternal medical conditions – such as cardiac disease or severe hypertension.

Some instrumental deliveries may need to be performed as an 'emergency' procedure e.g. a fetal bradycardia; some are performed in a more elective manner e.g. failure to progress in the second stage of labour with no fetal compromise. The instrument of choice is dependent on both maternal and fetal factors, and both instruments have a role.

Ventouse

There are three types of ventouse cup – the silastic, plastic and metal cups. They can be both disposable and non-disposable. They may need to be attached to a vacuum pump to generate negative pressure or may have an in-built system. The silastic/silk cups (Figure 8.4) are suitable for low pelvic cavity deliveries with good concomitant maternal effort. These are used to flex and guide the head and the operator cannot use significant effort to achieve delivery or the cup will simply detach off the fetal head. The metal cups are more robust and more difficult (including rotational) vaginal deliveries can be achieved.

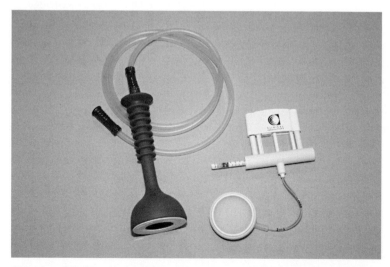

Figure 8.4 Disposable ventouse devices, on the right is a hand-held device with a hand-pump to generate suction via a hard plastic cup, on the left is a softer silicone-based cup, which is attached to suction via the tubing.

Advantages:
- Can be performed under pudendal/local anaesthetic with less maternal discomfort
- Do not increase the biparietal delivery diameter so an episiotomy may not be necessary
- Less maternal genital trauma

Disadvantages/Restrictions:
- More likely to fail to achieve delivery than with forceps
- More associated fetal trauma – scalp lacerations, retinal haemorrhages and cephalohaematoma
- Should not be used on fetuses under 35 weeks gestation

Forceps

Forceps can be used for non-rotational (numerous names e.g. Neville-Barnes, Simpson's) (Figure 8.5) and rotational deliveries (Kiellands). More operator effort can be exerted and these are often preferred for deliveries where the presenting part is in the mid-pelvic cavity, when there is no descent of the head from maternal effort or when there is caput and moulding present on the fetal head (which will lead to sub-optimal suction developing).

Advantages:
- More likely to achieve a vaginal delivery than with the ventouse
- Can be used if an instrumental delivery is needed in a premature baby

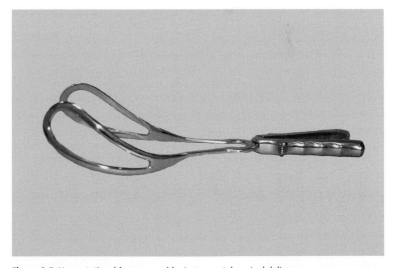

Figure 8.5 Non-rotational forceps used for instrumental vaginal delivery.

Disadvantages:
- More associated maternal genital trauma

To achieve a safe instrumental delivery using either instrument the following should be considered:[6]
- Less than 1/5th of the fetal head palpable abdominally
- Cephalic presentation
- Cervix is fully dilated and the membranes ruptured
- The position of the fetal head should be ascertained
- The mother should be fully counselled and consent (normally verbal) obtained
- Appropriate analgesia should be present – depending on the clinical situation and the maternal wishes
- Empty bladder
- Operator deemed to have the knowledge and skills or be appropriately supervised
- Back-up plan if vaginal delivery not achieved
- Personnel present at delivery trained in neonatal resuscitation
- Vaginal delivery should be abandoned if there is not progressive descent of the fetus with each pull or if delivery is not achieved over three contractions

Analgesia/anaesthesia required for instrumental delivery

In an emergency both ventouse and forceps can be performed under no additional analgesia. However, this will result in pain for the patient and measures should be taken to reduce this. In general a ventouse confers less additional pain to the delivery compared to forceps. If possible, all options should be discussed with the patient, to ensure she remains as pain free during the delivery as possible or as she requests. One must bear in mind that in emergency circumstances of acute fetal compromise, the obstetrician does not have time to ensure full and adequate analgesia. In these circumstances a delivery may need to be performed under as best analgesia as possible and the circumstances surrounding the delivery fully explained to the patient afterwards. Local anaesthetic such as lignocaine can be infiltrated into the perineum, or a pudendal block can be used. A pudendal block involves the administration of local anaesthetic using a specialised needle (Figure 8.6) over the path of the pudendal nerve as it passes near the ischial spine. This provides adequate anaesthesia for a forceps or ventouse delivery.

> #### Options for anaesthesia/analgesia for instrumental delivery
> - Perineal infiltration with local anaesthetic (there is an increased need for episiotomy with instrumental deliveries) (obstetrician/midwife)
> - Pudendal nerve blockade +/− perineal infiltration (obstetrician)
> - If *in situ*, epidural 'top-up' (midwife/anaesthetist)
> - Spinal analgesia in theatre (anaesthetist)

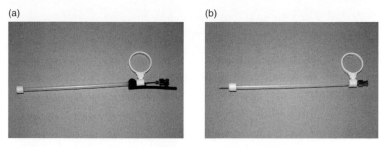

Figure 8.6 Pudendal needle used for administering a pudendal block. The needle is placed over the ischial spine while the protective cover remains in place; (a) when the needle is *in situ* the needle is introduced into the fascia surrounding the pudendal nerve (b) and local anaesthetic is administered.

Trial of vaginal delivery

This term is given to an attempted vaginal delivery that is considered to have a higher failure rate e.g. head at or just below the maternal ischial spines, fetal malpositions that will require an element of rotation to achieve delivery, maternal body mass index > 30, neonatal birthweight > 4 kg.[7] It is appropriate to conduct these deliveries in theatre. Consent will be informed; analgesia adequate (working epidural or spinal sited) and all personnel necessary present to perform an immediate Caesarean section should the attempt at vaginal delivery fail. This is a much more preferable situation (for mother, fetus and medical personnel) than failing to deliver the fetus in the room and needing to arrange to do a Caesarean section with no preparations in place.

Factors requiring trial of instrumental delivery in theatre:
- Requirement for rotational delivery (occipto-posterior/occipito-transverse position)
- High fetal head – at ischial spines
- Large baby/high index of suspicion of cephalo-pelvic disproportion

Anaesthesia for trial of instrumental vaginal delivery
- Anaesthesia should be adequate for immediate Caesarean section if vaginal delivery fails
- If epidural '*in situ*' – the top-up must be adequate for Caesarean section
- If no epidural, spinal anaesthesia is preferable – the same dose and drugs should be given as for a Caesarean section

> - If regional anaesthesia is contraindicated instrumental delivery should be attempted under pudendal nerve block, and the anaesthetist should be prepared to administer an immediate general anaesthetic if required

Complications of instrumental vaginal delivery

There are both fetal and maternal complications:

Maternal complications
- Failure to achieve delivery requiring abdominal delivery
- Genital trauma (including lateral vaginal wall tears, and third and fourth degree tears – see below)
- Postpartum haemorrhage (increased blood loss compared with spontaneous vaginal delivery, but less than a second stage Caesarean section)

Fetal complications
- Cephalohaematoma and scalp lacerations (ventouse)
- Retinal haemorrhages (ventouse)
- Forceps marks on the fetal face – normally transient
- Fractured skull (forceps)

Breech delivery

Breech presentation affects 3–4% of infants at term. It is more common in preterm deliveries.

Breech presentation is classified as follows (shown in Figure 8.7):
- Footling breech – the foot is the presenting part of the fetus (Figure 8.7a)
- Extended breech – the sacrum is the presenting part of the fetus. The hip is flexed and the knee is extended (Figure 8.7b)
- Flexed breech – the sacrum is the presenting part of the fetus. The hip and knee joints are both flexed (Figure 8.7c)

The perinatal outcome is worse for infants with breech presentation irrespective of mode of delivery. The risk of perinatal fetal death is reduced if infants are delivered by planned Caesarean section (Relative Risk 0.31).[8] This may result from fewer problems in delivery, including entrapment of the fetal head (when the fetal head cannot be delivered after the fetal body has already been delivered). The benefit of Caesarean section for infants is associated with an increased maternal morbidity.

Women with breech presentations at term (37–42 weeks) should be offered external cephalic version (ECV) unless contraindicated (intrauterine growth restriction (IUGR), fetal anomalies, low-lying placenta).[9] External cephalic version

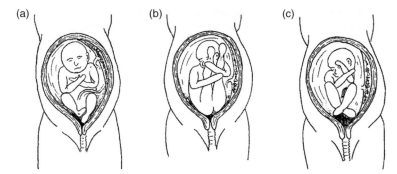

Figure 8.7 Breech presentations (a) Footling breech in which the fetal foot is the presenting part. (b) Extended breech, in which the fetal sacrum presents first, and the legs are extended. (c) Flexed breech, in which the fetal sacrum presents first and the legs are flexed at the knee.

is a procedure to rotate a breech presentation to a cephalic one. The fetal breech is disimpacted from the maternal pelvis and the baby rotated until it is cephalic. There is a higher success rate after 37 weeks gestation.

- ECV does not require anaesthesia, although may be more comfortable under regional anaesthesia
- Continuous fetal monitoring should be used before and after ECV
- Ultrasound assessment of the fetus is helpful
- ECV should be undertaken where emergency delivery can be performed if there are signs of fetal distress.
  Complications of ECV include:
- Fetal bradycardia in 10% of ECV (although it resolves spontaneously in most cases)
- Entanglement of umbilical cord
- Preterm labour
- Pre-labour rupture of membranes
- 0.9% risk of immediate Caesarean section

Anaesthetic implications of ECV:
- IV access should be obtained
- Immediate delivery by category 1 Caesarean section in < 1% of cases (usually by general anaesthesia if regional anaesthesia is not already in place)

The role of Caesarean section for delivery of breech presentations is less clear for multiparous women or women in labour. There is insufficient evidence to support

Caesarean section for preterm breech delivery. Footling breech should always be delivered by Caesarean section due to the risk of umbilical cord prolapse.

Obstetricians should remain familiar with the technique of assisted vaginal breech delivery, as some patients will present with breech presentation in preterm labour or in advanced labour when Caesarean delivery would be more difficult than assisted vaginal breech delivery. In addition, some patients prefer vaginal delivery to planned Caesarean section.

Assisted vaginal breech delivery

Assisted vaginal breech delivery should only take place in the absence of fetal and maternal contraindications (IUGR, macrocosmic fetus, no evidence of extension of the fetal head).

- Assisted vaginal breech delivery should be performed by a competent obstetrician.
- Excessive traction should not be applied to the fetus as this will cause extension of the fetal head, increasing the risk of head entrapment.
- Continuous fetal monitoring is required to detect fetal hypoxia.
- Regular vaginal examination is required. Nulliparous women should dilate at least 1 cm/hr, multiparous women at least 1.5 cm/hr.
- Second stage of labour should not last longer than 60 minutes.
- During the second stage when the presenting part descends onto the perineum the legs should be guided if necessary, by flexing the fetal knees.
- Further descent should be allowed, until the fetal pelvis is visible. The fetal back should be anterior, if this is not the case, the fetal pelvis should be rotated until the fetal spine is towards the maternal symphysis pubis.
- Further descent should occur with pushing, until the fetal scapulae are visible, the operator then rotates the fetus up to 180° in each direction to facilitate delivery of the arms.
- Further descent is then allowed until the fetal neck is visible; the operator should then deliver the fetus by flexion of the fetal head. This is best achieved with one hand on the fetal occiput and the other on the maxilla.
- Occasionally, the fetal head may be delivered using non-rotational forceps.

- Epidural analgesia is useful, but not essential for assisted vaginal breech delivery[10]
- Epidural analgesia reduces sensation and expulsive maternal efforts prior to full cervical dilatation. Delivery often needs manipulation of the fetus and episiotomy is usually performed – both of which are aided by good analgesia
- Failure to progress in labour, high presenting fetal part and fetal distress are indications for Caesarean delivery

Twin delivery

Twin pregnancies have a higher incidence of pre-term labour, IUGR and pre-eclampsia. The risk of preterm delivery is greater for monochorionic twins, which are also at risk of twin–twin transfusion syndrome. The aim of treatment is to continue twin pregnancies until term providing there is no evidence of maternal or fetal compromise.

If the leading twin is not cephalic twins should be delivered by Caesarean section. If the first twin is cephalic and the second twin is not a cephalic presentation, ECV can be performed after the delivery of the first twin, followed by artificial rupture of membranes to stabilise the fetal head in the pelvis. If this fails, internal podalic version can be performed and the obstetrician will then perform a vaginal breech delivery.

In labour
- Epidural analgesia is recommended.
- Low dose oxytocin infusion (2 miU/hr–32 miU/hr) may be required, especially after delivery of the first twin.
- The interval between delivery of monochorionic twins should be less than 30 minutes.
- There is no evidence to inform the optimal delivery interval of dichorionic twins providing there is no evidence of fetal compromise/hypoxia.
- Incidence of postpartum haemorrhage is increased following multiple pregnancy. Prophylactic oxytocin infusion (10 U/hr) may be given.

Perineal trauma

Repair of perineal trauma

Episiotomies do not routinely need to be performed during an instrumental vaginal delivery. When using a ventouse, there is no increased diameter to the biparietal diameter of the fetal head to be delivered and thus perineal trauma should not be increased compared to a normal vaginal delivery. However, in reality instrumental deliveries quicken the descent of the fetal head through the perineum, and thus natural stretching of tissues is not allowed and perineal trauma is increased. With forceps, there is an increase in diameter of the fetal head to be delivered and thus the rationale for performing an episiotomy is stronger. Women who have had a previous vaginal delivery will have had perineal tissue that has been stretched to some degree before, and thus in general their perineal trauma should be less. The definitions of perineal trauma (episiotomy layers to be repaired are the same as a 'second degree tear')[11] are shown in Table 8.1.

Table 8.1 Classification of perineal trauma

Degree	Trauma
First	Injury to the skin only
Second	Injury to the perineum involving perineal muscles but not involving the anal sphincter
Third	Injury to perineum involving the anal sphincter complex
	3a: less than 50% of external anal sphincter thickness torn
	3b: more than 50% of external anal sphincter thickness torn
	3c: involvement of the internal anal sphincter
Fourth	Injury to perineum involving the anal sphincter complex and anal epithelium

Some first and second degree tears are not sutured if haemostasis is already secured. Small randomised control trials have shown poorer wound healing if they are left unsutured and non-significant differences in short-term discomfort.[11] A Cochrane review has shown that absorbable synthetic material (e.g. rapid absorption polyglactin, e.g. Vicryl Rapide ™) is associated with less perineal pain and dehiscence as opposed to suturing with catgut – now withdrawn in the UK.[12] A Cochrane review has shown continuous subcuticular suture to the perineum to be associated with less short-term pain than interrupted sutures.[11] The important principles of repair are:[11]

- Suture as soon as possible after delivery to reduce bleeding/infection
- Good lighting is required
- Good anatomical alignment is required and consideration given to cosmetic results (if in doubt a more experienced person should be consulted)
- Rectal examination is required at the end of the procedure to ensure the suture material has not been inserted into the rectal mucosa

Third and fourth degree tears
The following factors are associated with an increased risk of a third or fourth degree tear:

- Birthweight over 4 kg
- Persistent occipito-posterior position
- Nulliparity
- Induction of labour
- Epidural analgesia
- Second stage longer than one hour
- Episiotomy
- Forceps delivery[13]

The prevalence of anal symptoms in women who have undergone third and fourth degree tear repair ranges from 25–57%. The correct recognition of these tears after delivery and correct environment for suturing with good technique is vital to reducing post-delivery symptoms.

It is recommended that repair of third and fourth degree tears is routinely carried out in theatre with adequate (preferably regional) anaesthesia. A pain-free and non-moving patient is essential to a good repair. This also provides adequate light, appropriate instruments and an assistant.[14] The use of broad-spectrum antibiotics intra-operatively and post-operatively is associated with less post-operative infection and wound dehiscence. Laxatives are also prescribed post-operatively to reduce wound dehiscence.[14]

The sphincter repair is usually performed first with monofilament sutures. The remainder of the tear is then sutured. All women should then be followed up by a gynaecologist, and if symptomatic referred to a colo-rectal surgeon for further investigations.

- Complex second, third or fourth degree tears should be repaired in the operating theatre
- Perineal trauma can cause postpartum haemorrhage – the patient should be adequately resuscitated if hypovolaemic
- The operator should be experienced
- The repair should be done promptly
- Preferred anaesthesia is spinal/epidural (if *in situ*)
- If third and fourth degree tear give broad-spectrum antibiotics
- Good post-operative analgesia
- Consider catheterisation

REFERENCES

1. Royal College of Obstetricians and Gynaecologists, The National Sentinel Caesarean Section Audit (London: RCOG Press, 2001).
2. National Collaborating Centre for Women's and Children's Health, *Caesarean Section Clinical Guidelines* (London: Royal College of Obstetricians and Gynaecologists, April 2004).
3. Royal College of Obstetricians and Gynaecologists, *Thromboembolic Disease in Pregnancy and the Puerperium*. Guideline Number 28 (London: RCOG Press, 2004).
4. Confidential Enquiry into Maternal and Child Health, *Why Mothers Die? 2000–2002 –* The Sixth Report of the Confidential Enquiries into Maternal Deaths in the United Kingdom (London: RCOG Press, 2004).
5. D. J. Rouse, C. Macpherson, M. Landon *et al.*, Blood transfusion and Caesarean delivery. *Obstet. Gynecol.*, **108**:4 (2006), 891–7.

6. Royal College of Obstetricians and Gynaecologists, *Operative Vaginal Delivery.* Guideline Number 26 (London: RCOG Press, 2004).

7. D. J. Murphy, R. F. Liebling, L. Verity, R. Swingler and R. Patel, Early maternal and neonatal morbidity associated with operative delivery in second stage of labour: a cohort study. *Lancet,* **358** (2001), 1203–7.

8. G. J. Hofmeyr and M. E. Hannah, Planned Caesarean section for term breech delivery. *Cochrane Database Syst. Rev.,* **3** (2003), CD000166.

9. M. Mushambi, External cephalic version: new interest and old concerns. *Int. J. Obstet. Anaesth.,* **10** (2001), 263–6.

10. Royal College of Obstetricians and Gynaecologists, *The Management of Breech Presentation.* Guideline Number 20b (London: RCOG Press, 2006).

11. Royal College of Obstetricians and Gynaecologists, *Methods and Materials used in Perineal Repair.* Guideline Number 23 (London: RCOG Press, 2004).

12. C. Kettle and R. B. Johanson, Absorbable synthetic versus catgut suture material for perineal repair. *Cochrane Database Syst. Rev.,* **2** (2000), CD000006.

13. C. Kettle and R. B. Johanson, Continuous versus interrupted sutures for perineal repair. *Cochrane Database Syst. Rev.,* **2**(2000), CD000947.

14. Royal College of Obstetricians and Gynecologists, *Third and Fourth Degree Perineal Tears Following Vaginal Delivery – Management.* Guideline Number 29 (London: RCOG Press, 2004).

FURTHER READING

Royal College of Obstetricians and Gynaecologists, *Thromboprophylaxis During Pregnancy, Labour and Delivery.* Guideline Number 37 (London: RCOG Press, 2004).

Obstetric haemorrhage

Alexander Heazell

Introduction

Obstetric haemorrhage is classified with respect to the birth of the infant; ante-partum haemorrhage (APH) describes any bleeding pv between the beginning of the 24th week of pregnancy and the delivery of the infant and postpartum haemorrhage (PPH) describes excessive blood loss following delivery. Obstetric haemorrhage may result in massive blood loss endangering the life of the mother, and the infant in the case of antepartum haemorrhage. In the Confidential Enquiry into Maternal and Child Health (CEMACH) 2000–2002, there were 17 maternal deaths directly attributed to haemorrhage.[1] The CEMACH recommends that all obstetric units have a protocol for the management of obstetric haemorrhage; all individuals working in delivery units should be familiar with local guidelines.[1]

Antepartum haemorrhage (APH)

Antepartum haemorrhage is defined as any vaginal bleeding after 24 weeks' gestation. It is a major cause of perinatal morbidity and mortality, including an increased risk of premature delivery. To a lesser extent APH increases maternal morbidity as a result of hospitalisation, operative intervention and coagulopathy. Rare causes of APH include cervical inflammation, cervical polyp, cervical cancer and vaginal trauma. Blood lost due to these causes is from maternal origin and is usually not significant. The four major causes of APH are:

- Placental abruption
- Placenta praevia
- Uterine scar dehiscence
- Vasa praevia

Placental abruption

Definition
Placental abruption describes premature separation of the placenta from the uterine wall; this may be partial or complete separation and can occur at any stage of pregnancy.

Associations
Placental abruption affects 1–2% of pregnancies and has an increased incidence in patients who are hypertensive, smokers, cocaine users, women with overdistension

Obstetrics for Anaesthetists, ed. Alexander Heazell and John Clift. Published by Cambridge University Press. © Cambridge University Press 2008

of the uterus (multiple pregnancy, polyhydramnios) and patients with a history of abdominal trauma.[2,3]

Presentation

Placental abruption may be *revealed* where there is bleeding pv (80% of cases) or *concealed* where there is no bleeding pv (20%). The amount of external bleeding does not correlate with total blood loss. Bleeding behind the placenta causes myometrial irritation, leading to abdominal pain. In the case of a small abruption this myometrial irritability may lead to the onset of labour; in the case of a large abruption the uterus will become hypertonic.

On examination, patients have tenderness of the uterus in the absence of uterine contractions; if there is a large abruption and uterine hypertonia the uterus will be hard and tense (classically described as "woody") and may be larger than expected for gestational age.

> Patients may not show any evidence of hypovolaemia, or may show signs of shock disproportionate to the observed blood loss due to the blood concealed within the uterus.

Initial sequelae

The initial blood loss from the placenta is maternal, however fetal blood volume may be reduced by trans-placental haemorrhage. The detached placenta is no longer able to function, therefore the fetus may become hypoxic and acidaemic, and is at increased risk of intrauterine fetal death (IUFD).[4]

Intervention

The intervention following placental abruption is dependent upon the severity of the abruption and the presence of fetal compromise. All Rhesus negative women should receive Anti-D with every episode of bleeding.[5] If the abruption is mild and the fetal heart rate is normal, the patient should be admitted for observation as the bleeding may cease. In moderate and severe abruption, the priority of treatment is resuscitation of the mother. Any further intervention will depend on whether the fetus is alive or dead. Basic management of moderate to severe abruption will always include:

- Airway, Breathing, Circulation
- Large-bore IV cannulae × 2
- Urinary catheter
- FBC, clotting studies
- Blood cross-match 6 units
- Correct coagulopathy with FFP/cryoprecipitate
- Assessment of fetal heart rate

- If the fetus is *alive* and *not compromised*, vaginal delivery may be possible. Labour should be induced by amniotomy (if membranes are still intact) and augmented with oxytocin while continually monitoring fetal heart rate.

In the case of vaginal delivery, epidural analgesia is the analgesia of choice.

- If the fetus is *alive* and *compromised* immediate delivery by Caesarean section is indicated.
- If the fetus has died vaginal delivery should be planned unless there is another obstetric indication for a Caesarean section such as transverse lie or the maternal haemorrhage is such that hypovolaemia and shock are uncontrollable.

General anaesthetic for Caesarean section should be considered if:
- It is an emergency Caesarean section requiring immediate delivery
- The patient is haemodynamically compromised
- Coagulopathy or Disseminated Intravascular Coagulation (DIC) are present

Postpartum sequelae
- Placental abruption is a risk factor for PPH (Relative risk of 2)

In placental abruption this may result from coagulopathy secondary to clotting factor consumption or from a 'Couvelaire' uterus, which describes the appearance of a pale uterus with black areas of intramyometrial blood, this myometrium is unable to contract effectively, leaving the placental bed vessels open. Agents that increase uterine contraction such as oxytocin and carboprost are used to increase uterine tone. If these fail to control the bleeding a hysterectomy may be required.

Complications may arise from blood loss, consumption of clotting factors and transfusion of large amounts of blood products.

If there are any maternal complications intra-operatively or post-operatively, the patient should be managed in a high-dependency area.

Placenta praevia

Definition
Placenta praevia describes a low-lying placenta that partially or wholly covers the internal cervical os. There are four different grades of placenta praevia (Figure 9.1).

Associations
Placenta praevia affects 0.5% of pregnancies. Ultrasound screening identifies many cases, 5–6% of patients will have a 'low-lying' placenta at 20 weeks gestation.

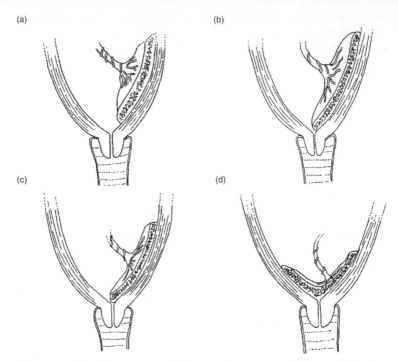

(a)   (b)

(c)   (d)

Figure 9.1 Grades of placenta praevia (a) Placenta in lower segment (b) Placental edge abuts but does not cover cervix (c) Placenta partially covers internal os (d) Placenta completely covers internal os.

The majority resolve due to anatomical changes to the lower segment in the third trimester. Placenta praevia is associated with a low site of placental implantation, which may occur in a previous Caesarean section scar.

Presentation

Placenta praevia presents with painless APH in the absence of labour. The blood lost is maternal and does not cause myometrial irritation. The initial episode of bleeding may be termed a 'sentinel bleed' as a small bleed may precede a larger haemorrhage. As the placenta occupies the lower portion of the uterus, the fetal head cannot engage, resulting in an increased incidence of abnormal lie.

If placenta praevia is suspected a digital examination *should not* be performed except in the operating theatre, as this could further disrupt the placenta and increase bleeding.

Initial sequelae

The initial blood loss from the placenta is maternal, however fetal blood volume may be reduced by trans-placental haemorrhage.

Intervention

The intervention following suspected placental praevia is dependent upon the severity of the bleeding and the location of the placenta. Grade 1 and 2 placenta praevia can have a vaginal delivery providing the placenta is not within 2 cm of the internal os.[6] All Rhesus negative women should receive Anti-D with every episode of bleeding.[5]

Mild bleeding with no evidence of hypovolaemia or fetal compromise
- Admit for observation
- Perform an ultrasound scan to localise the placenta (if not done already)
- Aim to prolong the pregnancy until at least 37 weeks
- Treat anaemia with iron replacement
- The patient should remain in an appropriately equipped unit
- Large-bore IV access at all times
- Cross-matched blood always available

Moderate to severe bleeding not responding to expectant management
In moderate and severe haemorrhage, the priority of treatment is resuscitation of the mother. There is no role for vaginal delivery in patients with Grade 3 or 4 placenta praevia. The acute management is the same as for severe abruption:
- Airway, Breathing, Circulation
- Large-bore IV cannulae × 2
- Urinary catheter
- FBC, clotting studies
- Blood cross-match 6 units
- Correct coagulopathy with FFP/cryoprecipitate
- Assessment of fetal heart rate

Invasive monitoring should be considered if the patient is haemodynamically unstable
If a large blood loss is expected, invasive monitoring, fluid warmers and patient-warming devices should all be considered.

Delivery is by Caesarean section for which cross-matched blood should be available for planned Caesarean sections. In the case of emergency Caesarean section, if cross-matched blood is unavailable, O Negative or type-specific blood should be used in the interim. Caesarean section for placenta praevia is associated with a greater blood loss compared to elective Caesarean section. Anterior placenta praevia, maternal age > 35 years and previous Caesarean section are associated with an increased intra-operative blood loss.

General anaesthetic for Caesarean section should be considered if:
- The patient is haemodynamically compromised
- Coagulopathy or DIC are present
- Massive blood loss is expected (e.g. anterior placenta praevia)

Otherwise regional anaesthesia is the technique of choice and associated with a reduced blood loss.

A **combined spinal epidural** may be considered if the surgery is expected to outlast a single-shot spinal block.

The large placental bed vessels lie in the lower segment in placenta praevia; this predisposes the patient to a PPH. Oxytocin or carboprost may be required to enhance uterine contraction, closing the myometrial vessels. If this is unsuccessful, hysterectomy may be required to control bleeding. Consent for hysterectomy should be obtained from women undergoing Caesarean section for placenta praevia. If there is significant blood loss and haemodynamic instability, patients should be monitored in a high-dependency area, and have their urea and electrolytes and haematological parameters checked.

If there are any maternal complications intra-operatively or post-operatively, the patient should be managed in a high-dependency area.

Uterine scar dehiscence/uterine rupture

Definition
Uterine scar dehiscence refers to any disruption of a uterine scar, which may occur during pregnancy or labour. Uterine rupture describes a spontaneous rupture of the uterus in the absence of a uterine scar.

Associations
Uterine scar rupture is reported in 0.3–1.7% of women with a uterine scar.[7] The most common uterine scar is lower segment Caesarean section, the risk is increased by repeated Caesarean section, and classical Caesarean section. There is an increased risk with surgical procedures resulting in a scar through all layers of the uterus such as myomectomy (removal of fibroids). Uterine rupture may occur following prolonged labour (particularly in the presence of oxytocin stimulation).

Presentation

Uterine scar dehiscence may be asymptomatic and discovered at elective Caesarean section. Symptoms may include bleeding pv or abdominal pain. Due to the proximity of the bladder to the lower segment of the uterus, haematuria may also be present. If dehiscence occurs during labour contractions may cease. On examination, there may be tenderness of the uterine scar, if there is complete dehiscence fetal parts may be palpable in the abdomen. The fetal heart rate trace may become abnormal after scar dehiscence. Patients may show sudden evidence of hypovolaemia.

Uterine rupture may present with pain, abnormalities of the fetal heart rate, or palpable fetal parts within the abdomen.

> Pain from uterine scar dehiscence and uterine rupture *can* be felt through low-dose epidural analgesia.

Initial sequelae

The initial blood loss from the uterus in uterine scar dehiscence is maternal. Placental function may be compromised and the fetus may become hypoxic and acidaemic. In the case of uterine rupture, the fetus will become immediately compromised.

Intervention

Following suspected uterine dehiscence or rupture the mother should be resuscitated. The fetus should be delivered by immediate Caesarean section; general anaesthesia is indicated due to the urgency of delivery. If the patient was receiving oxytocin to augment labour this should be immediately discontinued. Basic management will always include:

- Airway, Breathing, Circulation
- Large-bore IV cannulae × 2
- Urinary catheter (check for haematuria)
- FBC, clotting studies, blood cross-match 6 units
- Assessment of fetal heart rate

> **Invasive monitoring** should be considered if the patient is haemodynamically unstable.

> **General anaesthetic** for Caesarean section should be considered if:
> - Immediate delivery is required
> - The patient is haemodynamically compromised

Postpartum sequelae

Uterine scar dehiscence may be associated with damage to the urinary bladder. Caesarean section should include a careful assessment of the urinary tract. If the uterus cannot be repaired, then a hysterectomy may be performed.

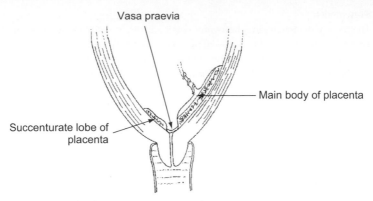

Figure 9.2 Vasa praevia showing fetal blood vessels in membranes from succenturate placental lobe.

Vasa praevia

Definition
Vasa praevia describes bleeding from fetal blood vessels that are present in the fetal membranes. All the blood loss is fetal (Figure 9.2).

Associations
Vasa praevia affects < 0.1% of pregnancies, it is associated with a low-lying placenta and a succenturate lobe, which describes a lobe of placenta separate from the main placental mass joined by vessels running along the membranes.[8]

Presentation
Vasa praevia presents with painless APH that is linked with spontaneous or artificial rupture of membranes. The blood lost is fetal, and associated changes in the fetal heart rate may be seen. Improvements in colour Doppler ultrasound have been able to identify fetal vessels lying adjacent to the cervix.[9]

Initial sequelae
The perinatal mortality rate is reported to be 50%. The blood loss is fetal, given that the blood volume of the newborn is approximately 75 ml/kg, the main risk is from fetal exsanguination.

Intervention
The intervention following suspected vasa praevia is immediate delivery by Caesarean section, under general anaesthesia due to the urgency of delivery. The infant may require volume replacement following delivery.

General anaesthetic for Caesarean section should be considered as immediate delivery is required to prevent fetal exsanguination.

Postpartum haemorrhage (PPH)

Definition

Postpartum haemorrhage (PPH) is defined as a blood loss greater than 500 ml in the first 24 hours after delivery or 1000 ml after Caesarean section. However, due to the lack of accuracy in predicting blood loss a more clinical definition is blood loss that produces haemodynamic instability.

Associations

PPH is associated with any problem that predisposes to coagulopathy or uterine atony, including:

Antepartum factors

- Pre-eclampsia
- Nulliparity
- Multiple gestation
- Previous PPH
- Previous CS

Intrapartum factors

- Prolonged labour
- Instrumental delivery
- Shoulder dystocia
- Prolonged third stage
- Oxytocin augmentation

Presentation

PPH presents with excessive blood loss following delivery of the infant, and may be massive. The patient may show symptoms of hypovolaemia.

Intervention

The management of PPH relies on rapid assessment of the cause and appropriate treatment to treat the bleeding. The most common causes of PPH are listed below in the order of frequency:

- Uterine atony
- Retained tissue
- Genital tract trauma
- Clotting disorders
- Uterine inversion

Primary treatment should concentrate on basic measures.

- Airway, Breathing, Circulation
- Large-bore IV cannulae × 2 (14 or 16 G)
- Urinary catheter (to deflate the bladder, and to record urine output)
- FBC, clotting studies
- Blood cross-match 6 units – inform transfusion department of PPH

Irrespective of the cause of PPH – if the patient is haemodynamically unstable, suffered massive blood loss (> 1000 ml), shows any evidence of coagulopathy, the patient should be managed in a **high-dependency facility**.

Uterine atony

Following delivery of the placenta the uterus contracts, closing the large blood vessels. A reduction in uterine contraction results in PPH. If the uterus is atonic, initially the uterus should be compressed between one hand in the vagina and another on the anterior abdominal wall – termed bimanual uterine massage, forcing the large blood vessels closed. During this time drugs leading to sustained myometrial contraction should be given, these include:

- If not given already 1 ml of Syntometrine (except in pre-eclamptic patients)
- Oxytocin – a further 5 unit bolus can be given IV followed by an infusion of 10 units an hour for at least 4 hours.
- Carboprost – 250 µg given IM can be repeated every 15 minutes up to 8 doses
- Misoprostol – 600 µg given PR

If medical methods fail to prevent further haemorrhage surgical treatment is indicated. Previous CEMACH reports have highlighted that maternal death from PPH may result from delayed surgical intervention.[1] The most common procedures performed are:

- Ligation/embolisation of the internal iliac artery – this may be done via laparotomy or via arteriography
- B-lynch suture – a large suture is placed from the posterior aspect of the uterus to the lower segment anteriorly, compressing the myometrial vessels
- Hysterectomy

Retained tissue

If placental tissue is retained the uterus is unable to contract adequately, which leads to bleeding by the same mechanism as uterine atony. The treatment is to remove the tissue manually, digitally separating the placenta from the uterine wall. This is associated with an increased incidence of intrauterine infection and further bleeding. Patients should receive broad-spectrum antibiotics and have further cross-matched blood available.

Regional anaesthesia is the anaesthetic of choice for retained placental tissue, in the absence of evidence that the placenta is morbidly adherent.

Rarely, retained placental tissue may be due to a morbidly adherent placenta; this may be:

- Placenta accreta – the placenta is adherent to the myometrium
- Placenta increta – the placenta invades the myometrium

- Placenta percreta – the placenta has invaded the myometrium and penetrates the serosal surface

Placenta accreta may be removed manually providing there is not excessive blood loss; however, other forms of morbidly adherent placentae may require hysterectomy to control bleeding. If these are detected antenatally by ultrasound, delivery will usually be by planned Caesarean section, with consent for hysterectomy obtained from the patient.

Genital tract trauma

During vaginal delivery trauma to the genital tract may be spontaneous or as a result of episiotomy. Tears may occur in the cervix, vagina or perineum, all may bleed profusely due to the increased vascularity of the area. Tears of the cervix and high vaginal tears will require examination under anaesthesia and suturing. Perineal tears are classified as:

- First degree – involve only the epithelial surface
- Second degree – involve the skin, subcutaneous tissues and superficial perineal muscles
- Third degree – as above, but also involves the anal sphincter
- Fourth degree – as above, but also involves the rectal mucosa

First and second degree perineal tears are usually repaired under local anaesthetic. However large second degree, third and fourth degree tears require regional or general anaesthesia due to the complexity of the repair, of which regional anaesthesia is the technique of choice.[10]

Clotting disorders

It is uncommon for a clotting disorder to cause PPH; however, clotting disorders frequently complicate PPH from all causes. Clotting disorders can result from:

- Pregnancy-associated thrombocytopaenia
- Pre-eclampsia
- Sepsis
- IUFD

Management includes urgent assessment of the full blood count (platelets) and clotting studies (PT and APTT). If the PT or APTT are prolonged this should be treated using fresh frozen plasma and cryoprecipitate.

Uterine inversion

This is caused by excessive cord traction in the absence of uterine contraction – the traction inverts the uterus. Cardiovascular compromise is worsened by an increase in vagal tone, which may require anticholinergic drugs to treat the resulting bradycardia. The management of uterine inversion involves rapid replacement of the uterus, which can be achieved manually or by hydrostatic pressure using saline. Due to the discomfort of this procedure, anaesthesia is required. When the inversion is corrected the signs of shock usually resolve quickly.

The replacement of the uterus requires uterine relaxation, which may be achieved by the use of:
- volatile anaesthetic agents
- nitrates
- magnesium
- beta-agonists.

General anaesthesia with relaxation by volatile agents is the most proven anaesthetic technique to correct the inversion.

REFERENCES

1. Confidential Enquiry into Maternal and Child Health, *Why Mothers Die 2000–2002 – The Sixth Report of the Confidential Enquiries into Maternal Deaths in the United Kingdom* (London: RCOG Press, 2004).
2. K. Hladky, J. Yankowitz and W. F. Hansen, Placental abruption. *Obstet. Gynecol. Surv.*, **57**:5 (2002), 299–305.
3. P. Nash and P. Driscoll, ABC of major trauma. Trauma in pregnancy. *BMJ*, **301**:6758 (1990), 974–6.
4. C. V. Ananth, G. S. Berkowitz, D. A. Savitz and R. H. Lapinski, Placental abruption and adverse perinatal outcomes. *JAMA*, **282**:17 (1999), 1646–51.
5. Royal College of Obstetricians and Gynaecologists, *Use of Anti-D Immunoglobulin for Rh Prophylaxis*. Guideline Number 22 (London: RCOG Press, 2002).
6. L. W. Oppenheimer, D. Farine, J. W. Ritchie *et al.*, What is a low-lying placenta? *Am. J. Obstet. Gynecol.*, **165**:4 Pt 1 (1991), 1036–8.
7. M. G. Rosen, J. C. Dickinson and C. L. Westhoff, Vaginal birth after cesarean: a meta-analysis of morbidity and mortality. *Obstet. Gynecol.*, **77**:3 (1991), 465–70.
8. W. Lee, V. L. Lee, J. S. Kirk *et al.*, Vasa previa: prenatal diagnosis, natural evolution, and clinical outcome. *Obstet. Gynecol.*, **95**:4 (2000), 572–6.
9. H. Arts and J. van Eyck, Antenatal diagnosis of vasa previa by transvaginal color Doppler sonography. *Ultrasound Obstet. Gynecol.*, **3**:4 (1993), 276–8.
10. Royal College of Obstetricians and Gynaecologists, *Management of Third- and Fourth-Degree Perineal Tears*. Guideline Number 29 (London: RCOG Press, 2007).

FURTHER READING

Royal College of Obstetricians and Gynaecologists, *Placenta Praevia and Placenta Praevia Accreta: Diagnosis and Management*. Guideline Number 2 (London: RCOG Press, 2001).

Bleeding in the latter half of pregnancy. In M. Enkin, M. J. N. C. Keirse, J. P. Neilson, *et al. A Guide to Effective Care in Pregnancy and Childbirth*, 3rd edn (Oxford: Oxford University Press, 2000), pp. 178–184.

D. M. Levy, Anaesthesia for Caesarean section. *Continuing Education in Anaesthesia, Critical Care and Pain*, **1** (2001), 171–6.

D. C. Mayer and F. J. Spielman, Antepartum and postpartum haemorrhage. In D. H. Chestnut, ed., *Obstetric Anaesthesia* (St Louis: Mosby, 2001).

C. Thomas and T. Madej, Obstetric emergencies and the anaesthetist. *Continuing Education in Anaesthesia, Critical Care and Pain*, **2** (2002), 174–7.

Thromboembolic disorders of pregnancy

Mark Tindall

Introduction

Pulmonary embolism is the most common direct cause of maternal death in the UK.[1] Successive reports from the Confidential Enquiry into Maternal and Child Health (CEMACH) have highlighted failures in recognition of risk factors for venous thromboembolism (VTE) and provision of adequate prophylaxis. In addition, difficulty in diagnosis and providing adequate treatment also exist.

Venous thromboembolism (VTE)

Venous thromboembolism is a significant cause of mortality and morbidity in pregnancy. The incidence varies widely, probably a reflection of the difficulties in diagnosis in this patient group, but is in the region of 0.8 to 1 in 1000 in the UK,[2] between 2 and 5 times greater than in the non-pregnant population. VTE is more common in pregnancy due to:

- *Increased venous stasis*
  - High oestrogen levels increase venous distensibility and capacity
  - Increased plasma volume
  - Compression of IVC by gravid uterus
- *Hypercoagulability*
  - Increase in certain clotting factors – Von Willebrand factor, fibrinogen, factors I, II, VII, VIII, IX and X
  - Decrease in natural anticoagulants – protein S
  - Resistance to activated protein C
  - Reduced fibrinolytic activity

There are two different manifestations of VTE – Deep vein thrombosis (DVT) and pulmonary embolism (PE).

Deep vein thrombosis

Definition
DVTs are organised clots that occur in the venous system, usually in the large veins of the leg or pelvis.

Epidemiology
The exact incidence is unknown but is up to five times higher in pregnancy. There appears to be little difference between the three trimesters. A sharp increase of five

Obstetrics for Anaesthetists, ed. Alexander Heazell and John Clift. Published by Cambridge University Press. © Cambridge University Press 2008

fold occurs in the postpartum period.[3] The commonest sites are in the iliac and/or femoral veins[2] with isolated calf DVT being less common. There is a striking propensity for the left leg, the venous drainage of the left leg being more tortuous and the left common iliac vein being traversed by the right common iliac artery.[4]

Presentation
Many are asymptomatic. The classical signs and symptoms can sometimes be normal occurrences during pregnancy making the clinical diagnosis even more difficult.
- Unilateral oedema
- Leg pain
- Tenderness
- Warmth and erythema
- Lower abdominal pain
- Fever and raised WCC
- Discoloration

Clinical course
Some smaller clots located below the knee can resolve spontaneously with no adverse sequelae. The principle concern is that the clot may propagate and then embolise lodging in the pulmonary circulation (PE). The rate of embolism formation can be as high as 20%, ileo-femoral thrombi carrying the highest risk.

Pulmonary embolus (PE)

Definition
A PE is a clot that causes occlusion of an artery in the pulmonary circulation. The blockage can be caused by air, fat, amniotic fluid or blood clot. By far the commonest cause is a blood clot originating as a DVT in the lower limbs.

Epidemiology
The incidence of PE is around three times less than that of DVT. However, PE can be fatal, being the leading direct cause of maternal death in the UK during the triennium 2000–2 in which 24 such deaths occurred. DVTs from all sites can be responsible. Emboli originating in the pelvic, axillary or subclavian veins are most commonly implicated in the cases of fatal PE.[5]

Presentation
Asymptomatic and atypical presentations are not uncommon. The classical triad of haemoptysis, dyspnoea and chest pain occur in less than 20% of patients. Any of the following may occur:
- Pleuritic chest pain
- Chest wall tenderness

- Rales or wheeze
- Tachypnoea
- Tachycardia
- Diaphoresis
- S3 gallop rhythm or murmur
- Fever
- Cyanosis

Massive PE may present with the above or with cardiovascular collapse/arrest.

> ### Immediate management of the pregnant patient with suspected massive PE
>
> **A**irway
> **B**reathing
> **C**irculation
>
> If cardiac arrest has occurred, follow Adult Life Support Universal Algorithm (Appendix 1) with the following additional considerations:
>
> - Left lateral tilt
> - Peri-arrest Caesarean section may be necessary to optimise resuscitation
> - Thoracotomy may be necessary to remove thrombus
>
> If patient conscious:
>
> - Sit up, reassure
> - 100% oxygen via Hudson mask with reservoir
> - Large-bore IV access
> - Fluid boluses as necessary for hypotension
> - Commence IV heparin
> - Consider fibrinolytic agents (recombinant tissue plasminogen activator (rtPA))
>
> Further investigation to confirm the diagnosis can be done once stability has been achieved.

Diagnosis of VTE

The accurate diagnosis of VTE requires both clinical assessment and objective testing. Less than 50% of women with clinically suspected VTE have the diagnosis confirmed on objective testing.

The following should be performed promptly in any pregnant woman with suspected DVT or PE.

DVT

Ultrasound (compression or duplex) of the lower limbs is the investigation of choice.

PE

Bilateral leg ultrasound and a ventilation–perfusion (V/Q) scan. If the patient is pregnant at the time of examination, a perfusion scan may be performed first to minimise exposure to radiation.

The effectiveness of these tests is variable. If they are negative yet a high degree of clinical suspicion persists, anticoagulant treatment should be commenced and the investigations repeated. Spiral CT scan may also be used to identify PE, although may be reserved for women with equivocal V/Q result.

Treatment

Evidence for the management of VTE during pregnancy is lacking. Recommendations are mainly extrapolated from non-pregnant subjects. Deep vein thromboses in pregnancy will require treatment.

Low molecular weight heparin (LMWH) is the treatment of choice.[2]

- Equally or more effective in both DVT and PE than unfractionated heparin
- Lower risk of haemorrhagic complications
- Lower mortality
- Good safety profile in pregnancy
- Less thrombocytopenia and osteoporosis

In clinically suspected DVT or PE, treatment with LMWH should be given until the diagnosis is excluded

Maintenance anticoagulant treatment should be continued with LMWH throughout the pregnancy. Frequent monitoring is not necessary but anti-Xa activity should be measured to confirm appropriate dosing, the timing of which should be in accordance with local haematology protocols.

Warfarin should not be used in pregnancy due to teratogenic effects and risk of antepartum haemorrhage. Warfarin is not a contraindication to breast-feeding, and can be given in the postpartum period.

Prevention

Thromboprophylaxis during pregnancy and the puerperium

In response to the deficiencies highlighted by CEMACH, the Royal College of Obstetricians and Gynaecologists (RCOG) have published clinical guidelines, which are regularly updated.[6] However, there is a lack of RCT evidence for prophylaxis strategies in pregnancy.

Assessment of antenatal risk

The first step in prevention is to assess those patients who are most at risk. Not only is pregnancy itself a significant risk factor but there are many additional risk factors (see Table 10.1).

Table 10.1 Risk factors for venous thromboembolism in pregnancy and the puerperium

Pre-existing	New onset or transient
Previous VTE	Surgical procedure
Thrombophilia	Hyperemesis gravidarum
Age >35	Dehydration
Obesity (BMI >30)	Severe infection
Parity >4	Immobility (>4 days bed-rest)
Gross varicose veins	Pre-eclampsia
Paraplegia	Excessive blood loss
Sickle cell disease	Long-haul travel
Inflammatory disorders	Prolonged labour
Cardiac disease	Instrumental delivery
Myeloproliferative disorders	

Adapted from RCOG Thromboprophylaxis guideline, 2004.[6]

Table 10.2 Thrombophilias present in pregnancy

Congenital	Acquired
Antithrombin deficiency	Antiphospholipid syndrome
Protein C deficiency	Lupus anticoagulant
Factor V Leiden	Anticardiolipin antibodies
Prothrombin gene variant	

Adapted from RCOG Thromboprophylaxis guideline, 2004.[6]

The level of risk for each individual factor is difficult to quantify but it is clear that a combination will significantly increase the overall risk. High-risk women should have a prospective management plan implemented.

Previous VTE

Women who have had a previous VTE have a significantly increased risk of recurrence during pregnancy. The risk is higher if the woman has a known thrombophilia or if the event occurred in an unusual site (such as the axillary vein). A list of relevant thrombophilias is shown in Table 10.2. They should be carefully screened for both inherited and acquired thrombophilia, although pregnancy may affect some results.

Thromboprophylaxis

In addition to the RCOG guidelines and this handbook collaboration should exist at a local level between obstetric and haematology departments.

- Minimise immobilisation and avoid dehydration
- Graduated elastic compression stockings. Worn antenatally in high-risk patients and during hospitalisation.

Antenatal and postpartum (6 weeks) LMWH should be offered to:
- Recurrent VTE or previous VTE + thrombophilia
- Certain thrombophilias (even if no previous VTE)

Antenatal LMWH and 3–5 days postpartum:
- Three or more risk factors

Post-partum LMWH only:
- Two risk factors

Clinical judgement must be used with regard to the weighting of the individual risk factors. Obesity, age and previous VTE carry particularly high risk. It is important to consider that risk may change during the pregnancy and therefore should be reassessed during labour.

Timing and duration of thromboprophylaxis

In the antenatal period prophylaxis should be initiated as early as possible.

The prothrombotic changes are maximal immediately following delivery. Low molecular weight heparin should be continued throughout labour and delivery in women who have been receiving it antenatally.

Postpartum prophylaxis should be given as soon as possible after delivery providing there is no contraindication (haemorrhage). The pro thrombotic changes do not revert to normal until several weeks after delivery, therefore it is usual to continue for 6 weeks in high-risk patients, and 3–5 days in the lower-risk group.

Agents used for thromboprophylaxis

LMWH

They are as effective as unfractionated heparin in pregnancy. It is not necessary to monitor patients except in certain conditions such as antithrombin deficiency. Monitoring is achieved by measuring anti-Xa levels.

In the postpartum period no adverse effects have been demonstrated during breast-feeding. Prolonged use may be associated with osteoporosis.

Warfarin

Warfarin should be avoided especially between 6 and 12 weeks gestation. There is a strong association with teratogenesis, miscarriage, fetal and maternal haemorrhage, stillbirth and neurological problems in the baby. It is safe after delivery and during breast-feeding although it requires close monitoring. It also carries an increased risk of PPH.

Aspirin

Low-dose aspirin is safe in pregnancy and has been shown in the non-pregnant population to reduce the risk of VTE following major surgery. It may therefore have a role in certain at-risk patients who may not necessarily justify the use of antenatal heparin; there is insufficient evidence to demonstrate any benefit for this purpose.

Caesarean section

As with any surgical procedure, there is a further increased risk of VTE post Caesarean section (CS). Ten of the 24 deaths reported in the UK between 2000 and 2002 were in this category.[1] Anyone undergoing CS should undergo risk assessment:

Low risk – early mobilisation and rehydration
  • Elective CS, no other risk factors

Moderate risk – Thromboembolic device (TED) stockings and/or LMWH
  • Age >35
  • Obesity >80 kg
  • Parity 4 +
  • Labour >12 hours
  • Pre-eclampsia
  • Infection
  • Immobility
  • Major illness
  • Emergency CS in labour

High Risk – TED stockings and LMWH
  • Three or more moderate risk factors
  • Extended surgery
  • Previous history of VTE or thrombophilia

Anaesthetic considerations

Both the prophylaxis and treatment of VTE can potentially have implications on the provision of regional anaesthesia or analgesia during labour and delivery. The siting of a spinal or an epidural both risk producing an epidural haematoma in a patient on anticoagulants. The removal of an epidural catheter may also precipitate bleeding. Epidural haematoma, although rare, can have devastating consequences, with permanent neurological deficit.

The incidence of epidural haematoma has been estimated as 1 in 150 000 after epidural and 1 in 220 000 after spinal anaesthesia,[7] but no data specific to pregnancy exists. There have been a number of case reports of epidural haematoma following use of LMWH.

The timing of regional anaesthetic techniques is crucial in order to minimise the risk of haematoma. Accepted practice is as follows, local protocols may differ:[2]

- Following a **prophylactic** dose of LMWH, a regional technique should not be used for **12 hours**. If *in situ*, an epidural catheter should not be removed for 12 hours
- Following a **therapeutic** dose of LMWH, **24 hours** should elapse before a regional technique is employed
- Following a spinal or removal of an epidural catheter, the next prophylactic dose of LMWH should be given at least **4 hours** later

It may be necessary to discuss individual cases with a senior anaesthetist.

Amniotic fluid embolism (AFE)[8]

Amniotic fluid embolism is a rare form of thromboembolic disease in pregnancy. It is an obstetric emergency. It is thought that the process may be more similar to anaphylaxis than a true physical embolism.

Definition
Amniotic fluid, fetal cells, hair or debris enter the maternal circulation and cause cardiorespiratory collapse.

Pathophysiology
This is poorly understood but may be due to either an anaphylactic reaction or complement activation or both. There are thought to be two phases:
- Phase 1 – Pulmonary artery spasm, raised right heart pressures leading to hypoxia. Myocardial damage, left heart failure and acute respiratory distress syndrome.
- Phase 2 – Haemorrhagic. Uterine atony and consumptive coagulopathy with DIC.

Epidemiology
The incidence is approximately 1 in 8000 to 1 in 30 000 pregnancies.[8] In the UK between 2000 and 2002, 19 cases were reported.[1] Mortality has been quoted as high as 60–80%. However, in the UK cases (2000–2) mortality was 25%, although most survivors have significant neurological deficit. Fifty per cent of maternal mortality occurs in the first hour. Neonatal survival is 70%. Due to the rarity of this disorder there is little evidence to support definite associations and risk factors; hence it remains an unpredictable disease.

Clinical presentation

The onset usually occurs in the late stages of labour, but can occur during Caesarean section, abdominal trauma or abortion. It is a very acute sequence of events, with rapid progression, and may include:

- Acute dyspnoea
- Profound hypotension
- Seizures
- Cyanosis
- Pulmonary oedema
- Uterine atony
- Cardiac arrest
- Fetal bradycardia

> The diagnosis of AFE is a clinical one.
> Resuscitation should start as soon as symptoms present.

Management

Treatment is entirely supportive. There are no specific therapies.

- Airway – intubation often necessary. 100% oxygen
- Breathing
- Circulation – start CPR if cardiac arrest
- Fluids and inotropes for hypotension
- Invasive monitoring – arterial line, CVP line. A pulmonary artery catheter may be useful to assess filling pressures
- Correct coagulopathy – FFP, platelets, cryoprecipitate. Recombinant factor VIIa has been used with some success

If the AFE occurs before delivery, and is associated with cardiac arrest, perimortem Caesarean section should be performed after 4 minutes of cardiac arrest. Delivery of the baby will increase venous return to the heart, and decrease the proportion of cardiac output going to the uterus. (See Chapter 12.)

Admission to ITU will inevitably be required. Pulmonary oedema is common so fluid balance should be managed with care.

Following the acute event, histological findings may provide confirmatory evidence of the diagnosis of AFE. Fetal debris such as squamous cells and mucin may be aspirated from central venous blood and are frequently found in the pulmonary capillaries at post mortem.

Amniotic fluid embolism is a devastating condition which should always be considered if a woman collapses in labour or the puerperium. Early involvement of the anaesthetic team is important. The mortality may not be as high as once feared, therefore early recognition and treatment may be life saving.

Sudden obstetric collapse syndrome[9]

The traditional thinking regarding the cause and mechanism of AFE has long been questioned to the extent that it is believed by some parties to be misnamed. Yentis has proposed the term "Sudden Obstetric Collapse Syndrome", which reflects the clinical nature of the diagnosis in the absence of any significant evidence that amniotic fluid is actually the causative substance.[9] Amniotic fluid is not consistently harmful when infused into animals and humans nor is fetal debris always present in the pulmonary circulation.[9] The theory of an anaphylactic type reaction is debatable due to the low incidence of bronchospasm and relatively common occurrence of seizures.

It is clear that this condition is still very poorly understood, but early recognition and intervention remain of paramount importance.

REFERENCES

1. J. Drife, Thrombosis and thromboembolism. In Confidential Enquiry into Maternal and Child Health: *Why Mothers Die 2000–2002*. (London: RCOG Press, 2004) pp. 61–73.
2. Royal College of Obstetricians and Gynaecologists' *Thromboembolic Disease in Pregnancy and the Puerperium: Acute Management*. Guideline Number 28 (London: RCOG Press, 2001).
3. J. Heit, C. Kobbervig, A. James *et al.*, Trends in the incidence of venous thromboembolism during pregnancy or postpartum: a 30-year population-based study. *Ann. of Intern. Med.* **143**:10 (2005), 697–706.
4. A. Sumeja, Rashmi, M. Arora and N. Agarwal, Deep Vein Thrombosis (DVT) in Pregnancy. *J. Indian Acad. Clin. Med.*, **2**:4 (2001), 260–8.
5. C. Feied, Pulmonary embolism. *eMedicine* 2006. Available at www.emedicine.com.
6. Royal College of Obstetricians and Gynaecologists' *Thromboprophylaxis During Pregnancy, Labour and After Normal Vaginal Delivery*. Guideline Number 37 (London: RCOG Press, 2004).
7. M. Tryba, Spinal anaesthesia in the heparinised patient. *Int. Monitor Reg. Anaesth.*, **7**:4 (1995), 3–6.
8. L. Moore, Amniotic fluid embolism. *Emedicine* 2005. Available at emedicine.com.
9. S. M. Yentis, Sudden obstetric collapse syndrome. *Int. J. Obstet. Anesth.*, **8**:4 (1999), 296.

Infection

Paul Dias

Prophylaxis and Screening

Infection occurring in pregnancy can result in significant morbidity and mortality for both mother and child. Depending on the type of infection, there is an increased incidence of preterm delivery, intrauterine growth restriction, intrauterine and infant death and mother-to-child transmission of infection.

Screening is performed routinely for the following infections:

- Asymptomatic bacteriuria, by midstream urine culture. Treatment reduces the risk of maternal pyelonephritis and preterm birth.
- Serological screening of hepatitis B virus. Effective postnatal intervention reduces the risk of mother-to-child transmission in future pregnancies.
- Serological testing for HIV enables effective antenatal planning to reduce vertical transmission rates.
- Rubella-susceptibility screening enables postnatal vaccination to protect future pregnancies.
- Syphilis screening is also offered because treatment is beneficial to mother and fetus.

Pregnant women are advised of primary prevention measures to avoid contact with chickenpox (varicella-zoster virus), cytomegalovirus, *Toxoplasma* (cat litter/faeces) and *Listeria* (soft cheese/pate).

Planned Caesarean section for infection prophylaxis

A planned Caesarean section is recommended as an intervention in the following groups to reduce the risk of mother-to-child transmission:

- HIV-positive women who are not taking highly active antiretroviral therapy (HAART)
- HIV-positive women with a detectable viral load or low CD4 cell count
- Pregnant women who are co-infected with hepatitis C and HIV
- Women with primary genital herpes simplex virus infection occurring in the third trimester of pregnancy

Prophylaxis of infection related to obstetric procedures

Obstetric procedures such as Caesarean section, manual removal of placenta and 3rd degree tear repair are associated with a high rate of post-operative infection. To reduce the incidence of infection antibiotic prophylaxis is recommended at the time of surgery.

Obstetrics for Anaesthetists, ed. Alexander Heazell and John Clift. Published by Cambridge University Press. © Cambridge University Press 2008

All women having a Caesarean section should be offered prophylactic antibiotics, such as a single dose of first-generation cephalosporin or ampicillin and an agent to cover against anaerobes such as metronidazole, to reduce the risk of post-operative infections (such as endometritis, urinary tract and wound infection), which occur in about 8% of women who have had a Caesarean section.

Women undergoing repair of a third or fourth degree tear require intra-operative and post-operative antibiotic therapy to prevent infection which increases wound breakdown and the incidence of fistula formation. Intra-operatively, a broad-spectrum antibiotic such as a cephalosporin combined with an agent suitable to treat anaerobic organisms such as metronidazole should be given.

Chorioamnionitis

Chorioamnionitis is inflammation of the membranes that surround the fetus and the amniotic cavity. Ascending infection via ruptured membranes is the most common cause, especially following prolonged rupture of membranes or prolonged labour. However, transplacental transport can occur. Implicated pathogens include group B streptococci (GBS), *Escherichia coli* and *Bacteroides* sp.
- Symptoms may include fever, tachycardia, uterine tenderness and purulent/foul-smelling vaginal discharge.
- Maternal complications include postpartum infection and haemorrhage, sepsis and increased incidence of Caesarean section.
- Neonatal complications include pneumonia, meningitis, sepsis and death.
- Treatment is directed at an identified organism or with a second-third-generation cephalosporin. Gentamicin may be added in severe cases.
- Penicillin G is active against GBS. The recommended dose is 3 g intravenously followed by 1.5 g every 4 hours during labour. Intravenous clindamycin 900 mg 8 hourly should be administered to those who are penicillin allergic.

In Chorioamnionitis
- Broad-spectrum antibiotic therapy is started intrapartum (check local antibiotic policy) and continued post delivery
- Higher incidence of Caesarean section
- Regional anaesthesia and analgesia have not been shown to have an increased risk of complications

Group B streptococcus

Group B streptococcal infection is the most frequent cause of severe sepsis in the first week of life.

There is no screening programme for GBS in the UK, although approximately 25% of women may carry GBS. Group B streptococci may be detected in urine samples or vaginal swabs taken antenatally. Women with overt signs of infection e.g. urinary tract infection with GBS bacteriuria should receive appropriate treatment. In women who have GBS diagnosed incidentally (without signs of overt infection):

- Treatment is not recommended in the antenatal period or before labour
- Intrapartum treatment should be offered after discussion with the patient

Women who carry GBS and have a pyrexia $> 38\,°C$, prolonged rupture of membranes (> 18 hours), or premature labour are at increased risk of GBS.

- Intrapartum treatment should be offered after discussion with the patient
- If chorioamnionitis is present, treatment should include broad-spectrum antibiotics effective against GBS, rather than treatment for GBS alone.

Intrapartum treatment is with IV penicillin (clindamycin if allergic to penicillin). The Royal College of Obstetricians and Gynaecologists guidelines recommend a 3 g loading dose IV followed by 1.5 g every 4 hours until delivery. The first dose should be given at least 2 hours before delivery.

Women undergoing delivery by elective Caesarean section with intact membranes do not require antibiotic prophylaxis.

HIV and pregnancy

Introduction

Human immunodeficiency virus is a retrovirus that infects cells in the human immune system. There are three main routes of transmission (sexual, blood-borne and mother-to-child). Infection is associated with a progressive reduction in the $CD4^+$ T cell count. Following a latency period, the reduction in immune system function can lead to opportunistic infections, reactivation of latent viruses and appearance of certain tumours.

- Specific complications of HIV can result in chronic diarrhoea, drug-induced hepatitis, encephalopathy, neuropathy, dementia, nephropathy and pericarditis
- Treatment of women with high viral load usually consists of HAART to stabilise symptoms and reduce viraemia
- Recognised complications of certain HAART regimens include lactic acidosis, gastrointestinal disturbance, fatigue, fever and breathlessness

Implications for pregnancy

The risk of mother-to-child transmission is estimated to vary from 15–40%. The rate of transmission of HIV is dependent on maternal viral load, obstetric factors (vaginal delivery, prolonged rupture of membranes, chorioamnionitis and pre-term delivery) and breast-feeding. Effective interventions can reduce the risk of vertical transmission to less than 2%.

Antenatal care consists of screening and planned interventions to reduce the risk of mother-to-child transmission, which occurs largely in the third trimester:

- Antiretroviral therapy taken during pregnancy and delivery, even if normal CD4$^+$ count and low viral load
- Planned Caesarean section – the patient should be admitted for administration of IV high-dose zidovudine for 4 hours before delivery
- Avoidance of breast-feeding

Anaesthetic implications of HIV infection
- Universal precautions should be adhered to
- A maternal sample for viral load should be taken at delivery
- General anaesthesia is considered safe, but drug interactions and effects on organ systems should be assessed pre-operatively
- Regional anaesthesia is usually the technique of choice
- Local infections or specific complications may influence anaesthetic technique and should ideally be assessed by prenatal anaesthetic consultation

Timing of Caesarean section:
- A zidovudine infusion should be started 4 hours before the beginning of Caesarean section and continued until the cord is clamped
- This should be done after 38/40
- Although elective initially, once the infusion has been started the Caesarean section should NOT be delayed

Postpartum management
- In the UK all women who are HIV positive are advised not to breast-feed their babies
- Women requiring HAART for their own health (rather than that of their baby) should continue HAART
- Neonates should be treated with anti-retroviral therapy from birth

Genital herpes and pregnancy

Introduction
Genital herpes is a common cause of genital ulceration and is caused by herpes simplex virus type-1 (HSV-1) or herpes simplex virus type-2 (HSV-2).

- Transmission is by sexual intercourse or orogenital contact; commonly from an asymptomatic partner.
- After exposure symptoms may include genital pain, dysuria, fever and malaise. Genital erythema and painful ulceration develops typically 2 to 14 days post-exposure.

- Complications include dissemination, a short-lived meningitis and sacral autonomic and sensory disturbances (resulting in paraesthesia and urinary problems).
- Recurrent infections tend to be short-lived and less severe.
- Treatment is generally supportive (analgesia, help with urination). Acyclovir reduces the duration of symptoms and viral shedding.

Implications for pregnancy

- The risks to the neonate are greatest when a woman acquires a new infection during the third trimester.
- Neonatal herpes can occur as a result of direct contact with infected maternal secretions and can lead to a severe systemic viral infection with a high morbidity and mortality.
- There is an incidence of 1.65 per 100 000 live births annually in the UK.

Management of women presenting with their first episode of genital herpes in pregnancy

- Daily suppressive acyclovir in the last 4 weeks of pregnancy may prevent genital herpes recurrences at term
- Caesarean section is recommended for all women presenting with their first episode of genital herpes lesions at the time of delivery
- Those within 6 weeks of the expected delivery date or presentation with preterm labour may be considered for elective Caesarean section
- Invasive obstetric procedures e.g. fetal blood sampling should be avoided in those opting for a vaginal delivery
- Intravenous acyclovir given intrapartum to the mother and subsequently the neonate may reduce the risk of transmission

Management of women presenting with a recurrent episode of genital herpes during pregnancy

- A recurrent episode during the pregnancy is not an indication for Caesarean section
- The risks to the baby of neonatal herpes are small with recurrent lesions at the onset of labour and should be set against the risks of Caesarean section

Anaesthetic implications[1] of Genital Herpes

- Regional anaesthetic techniques are considered safe with recurrent genital herpes in the absence of systemic infection.
- With primary infection the patient may be viraemic. The theoretical risk of CNS infection must be weighed against the risks of providing alternative methods of anaesthesia and analgesia.

REFERENCE

1. A. M. Bader, W. R. Camann and S. Datta, Anesthesia for Caesarean delivery in patients with herpes simplex virus type-2 infections. *Reg. Anesth.*, **15**:5 (1990 Sep–Oct), 261–3.

FURTHER READING

National Institute for Health and Clinical Excellence. *Antenatal care: routine care for the healthy pregnant woman*. Clinical Guideline. (London: Department of Health, 2003).

Royal College of Obstetricians and Gynaecologists, *Management of Genital Herpes in Pregnancy*. Guideline Number 30 (London: RCOG Press, 2002).

Royal College of Obstetricians and Gynaecologists, *Management of HIV in Pregnancy*. Guideline Number 39 (London: RCOG Press, 2004).

Royal College of Obstetricians and Gynaecologists, *Prevention of Group B Streptococcal Infection*. Guideline Number 36 (London: RCOG Press, 2005).

Life support in obstetrics

Julian Chilvers

Introduction

Cardiac arrest in pregnancy is an extremely rare occurrence. It is very difficult to estimate the exact incidence as successful outcomes are rarely reported. Rees suggested the incidence was approximately 1 in 30 000 of late pregnancies.[1] This figure may be an underestimate if we consider the incidence of maternal deaths in pregnancy in the UK during the triennium 2000–2 is 13.1 per 100 000 pregnancies.[2]

Causes

As well as the causes of cardiac arrest for non-pregnant females of this age group e.g. trauma, anaphylaxis and drug overdose, there are a number of causes specific to the pregnant female, shown in Table 12.1.

Other possible scenarios include iatrogenic causes such as:

- Local anaesthetic toxicity
- Total spinal
- Hypermagnesaemia
- Hypoxaemia from a failed intubation

Intervention

Effective resuscitation of the mother is the most effective way to optimise fetal outcome. Resuscitation attempts should follow the Resuscitation Council (UK) guidelines on advance life support (see Appendix 1); however, these need to be modified when dealing with a pregnant mother.

- **Airway**

  Early intubation is necessary to minimise the risk of reflux due to a lax lower oesophageal sphincter.

  The anaesthetist should be prepared for a difficult intubation owing to airway oedema and engorged breasts making placement of the laryngoscope more challenging.

- **Breathing**

  The functional residual capacity is reduced in the pregnant mother leading to a tendency for the patient to desaturate more rapidly. Higher airway pressures may also be experienced owing to the raised intra-abdominal pressure.

Obstetrics for Anaesthetists, ed. Alexander Heazell and John Clift. Published by Cambridge University Press. © Cambridge University Press 2008

Table 12.1 Causes of maternal death investigated by confidential enquiry into maternal deaths 2000–2

	Number of deaths (2000–2)[2]
Pre-existing cardiac disease	44
Thromboembolism	30
Haemorrhage	17
Suicide/psychiatric illness	16
Hypertensive disorders of pregnancy	14
Ectopic pregnancy	11
Infection and sepsis	11
Amniotic fluid embolism	5

- **Circulation**

> At a gestational age of 20 weeks and beyond, the pregnant uterus can press against the inferior vena cava and aorta, impeding venous return and reduce the cardiac output by up to 70%.

The patient must be placed in an inclined lateral position to displace the uterus. This can be achieved by:
- Cardiff Wedge
- Pillow/blanket
- Manual displacement of the uterus

The full lateral position is not appropriate as it would not be possible to perform effective chest compressions in this position.

Chest compressions should be performed slightly higher than in a non-pregnant patient due to the elevation of the diaphragm and abdominal contents caused by the gravid uterus.

If the mother requires defibrillating, the same energy levels should be used as with a non-pregnant patient. Nanson demonstrated there is no statistically significant difference in transthoracic impedance in the pregnant and non-pregnant patient as originally thought.[3]

If hypermagnesaemia is suspected, consider treating with 10% calcium gluconate.

Perimortem Caesarean section

The greatest chance for both mother and baby to survive during a cardiac arrest is if the baby is delivered in order to relieve the aortocaval compression. This also allows for full resuscitation of the baby.

Table 12.2 The influence of gestational age on the indication for perimortem Caesarean section

Gestational age	Intervention
< 20 weeks	Perimortem CS unnecessary
20–24 weeks	Performing a perimortem CS will improve the chances of survival for the mother, but the baby is not viable at this age
> 24 weeks	Performing a perimortem CS will improve the chances of survival for the mother and baby

In a mother who is greater than 20 weeks gestation, a perimortem CS should be performed after 4 to 5 minutes of a cardiac arrest if there is no restoration of a spontaneous output.

Incidence
The incidence of perimortem CS in the UK is quoted as 1 in every 170 000 deliveries.[4] The decision to proceed to perimortem CS is dependent on gestation; outline guidance is shown in Table 12.2. In all instances perimortem CS is carried out primarily to improve survival of the mother.

Timing
There have been the occasional case reports showing neonatal survival after 15–20 minutes of cardiopulmonary resuscitation.[5,6] However it is well recognised that irreversible brain and tissue damage due to hypoxia occurs around 4–6 minutes.[7] Therefore a limit of 5 minutes is taken as the time by which the baby should have been delivered. The importance of adherence to this guideline is exemplified by the data in the 2000–2 Confidential Enquiry into Maternal and Child Health report, that 8 out of 19 babies survived a perimortem CS.[2]

In reality, in order for this time limit to be met, preparation for a perimortem CS should be made immediately on commencing resuscitation. Factors that increase the chance of the baby's survival at a perimortem CS are:[8]
- Short interval between mother's arrest and infant's delivery
- No sustained pre-arrest hypoxia in the mother
- No signs of fetal distress before the mother's arrest
- Aggressive and effective resuscitation

Procedure
It has been recommended that a classical midline approach should be used to speed up the procedure as there is natural diastasis of the recti muscles in late

pregnancy. However using a familiar procedure such as the lower segment approach may be just as rapid assuming that the operator will be experienced in this approach.

REFERENCES

1. G. A. D. Rees and B. A. Willis, Resuscitation in late pregnancy. *Anaesthesia*, **43** (1988), 347–9.
2. Confidential Enquiry into Maternal and Child Health, *Why Mothers Die 2000–2002 –* The Sixth Report of the Confidential Enquiries into Maternal Deaths in the UK (London: RCOG Press, 2004).
3. J. Nanson, D. Elcock, M. Williams and C. D. Deakin, Do physiological changes in pregnancy change defibrillation energy requirements? *Br. J. Anaesth.*, **87** (2001), 237–9.
4. M. Whitley and L. Irvine, Postmortem and perimortem Caesarean section: what are the indicators? *J. R. Soc. Med.*, **93** (2000), 6–9.
5. H. F. Chen, C. N. Lee, G. D. Hwang *et al.* Delayed maternal death after perimortem Caesarean section. *Acta Obstet. Gynecol. Scand.*, **73** (1994), 939–41.
6. J. A. Lopez-Zeno, W. A. Carlo, J. P. O'Grady and A. A. Fanaroff, Infant survival following delayed postmortem Caesarean delivery. *Obstet. Gynecol.*, **76** (1990), 991–2.
7. A. Page-Rodriguez and J. Ganzalez Sanchez, Perimortem Caesarean section of twin pregnancy. *Acad. Emerg. Med.*, **10** (1999), 1072–4.
8. American Heart Association, Supplement. Part 10.8: Cardiac arrest associated with pregnancy. *Circulation*, **112**:IV (2005), 150–3.

FURTHER READING

S. Morris and M. Stacey, ABC of resuscitation: resuscitation in pregnancy. *BMJ*, **327** (2003), 1277–9.

J. Nolan, J. Soar, A. Lockey, *et al.* (eds.) Adult *Advance Life Support*, 5th edn (London: Resuscitation Council (UK), 2005).

Drugs in obstetrics

Lisa Penny

Introduction

Drugs used in obstetrics merit special mention because they have their effects on two patients rather than one. Pharmacologically they are of particular interest because they may be transferred across, and metabolised by, another organ, the placenta. It is important for the anaesthetist to have an understanding of the drugs commonly used by obstetricians, the evidence for them and their interface with anaesthetics.

Drugs to increase uterine contractions

Indications
- Acceleration/augmentation of labour
- To minimise risk of postpartum haemorrhage (PPH)
- Treatment of PPH

Oxytocin
- In the UK a synthetic oxytocin is manufactured under the name syntocinion. It is a nonapeptide used to induce and augment labour and also to minimise blood loss post-delivery.
- It is thought to act by binding to myometrial cell receptors and increasing smooth muscle contractility.
- Guidelines from the Royal College of Obstetricians and Gynaecologists recommend that to induce or accelerate labour, oxytocin is given intravenously starting at a rate of 1–2 miU/min, titrated to uterine contractions and increasing every 30 minutes to a maximum of 32 miU/min.[1]
- It may also be given as a dose of 5 units slowly after delivery of baby during Caesarean section.
- Can be given as an infusion of 10 U/hr for the treatment prevention of PPH secondary to uterine atony. This is normally for a period of 4 hours.
- Its main adverse effect is the relaxation of vascular smooth muscle causing hypotension and a reflex tachycardia: this is potentiated in vasoconstricted states such as pre-eclampsia and hypovolaemia. It also has an antidiuretic effect, which can lead to water intoxication in large doses. Other side effects include nausea, vomiting and rashes.

Obstetrics for Anaesthetists, ed. Alexander Heazell and John Clift. Published by Cambridge University Press. © Cambridge University Press 2008

Ergometrine

- It is used to treat post-partum uterine atony and bleeding.
- It has a direct action on uterine smooth muscle via alpha-adrenergic pathways, increasing muscle tone and contractile frequency.
- It is rapidly absorbed after IM administration at a dose of 500 µg.
- The adverse effects include profound hypertension, especially in patients with pre-eclampsia or pre-existing high blood pressure. Bradycardia, myocardial ischaemia and acute heart failure may also occur; there is a particular danger if given in combination with an alpha-agonist such as methoxamine. Its gastrointestinal effects include nausea and increased lower oesophageal sphincter pressure.

Syntometrine is a combination of 500 µg ergometrine with oxytocin 5 Units.

Anaesthetic implications

- After delivery of baby, to cause uterine contraction at Caesarean section, oxytocin 5 units is given slowly to avoid hypotension
- After Caesarean section an oxytocin infusion may be given at 10 U/hr to prevent PPH
- During Caesarean section, ergometrine is avoided, if possible, because of the nausea and vomiting it causes
- Ergometrine and Syntometrine are usually avoided in patients with hypertension or pre-eclampsia unless there is severe PPH

Prostaglandins

Prostaglandin E_2 (dinoprostone)

- Used for cervical ripening during induction of labour (IOL).
- Kept at 4 °C in refrigerator.
- National Institute for Health and Clinical Excellence (NICE) guidelines suggest that prostaglandins should be used in preference to oxytocin for IOL when the membranes are intact. Both are equally effective when the membranes have ruptured.[1]
- Mediated by cyclo-oxygenase pathway receptors.
- Can be administered by vaginal route. The oral route is no longer used because of the adverse gastrointestinal side effects such as nausea, vomiting and diarrhoea. The NICE guidelines suggest that intravaginal prostaglandin E_2 (PGE_2) should be used rather than the intracervical route because it is equally effective but less invasive.
- NICE guidelines recommend nulliparous women receive Vaginal PGE_2 as either 3 mg tablets which can be repeated after 6 hours or 2 mg gel supplemented with a further 1 mg after 6–8 hours.[1]
- Side effects include maternal discomfort from the contractions and uterine hyperstimulation, which can compromise the fetus.

Prostaglandin E$_1$ (misoprostol)
- Synthetic PGE$_1$ analogue.
- Kept at room temperature.
- There is well-established evidence for its use in IOL, cervical ripening and in the prevention and management of PPH. It is not approved for these indications in most countries, including the UK.
- The dose varies with indication; for IOL, 25 µg vaginally has been used in primigravidae.
- Side effects include pyrexia, abdominal pain and nausea and vomiting. It has rarely been associated with uterine rupture. May lead to more uterine hyper-stimulation than PGE$_2$ analogues.
- For the prevention and/or treatment of PPH, a dose of 600–1000 µg po or pr can be used.[2,3,4,5] However, there is insufficient evidence to recommend misoprostol for the prevention of PPH at this time.
- The most effective dose of misoprostol for the treatment of PPH is between 800 and 1000 µg pr.

Carboprost
- Synthetic analogue of PGF$_{2\alpha}$.
- Kept at 4 °C in refrigerator.
- Indication: to treat PPH after failure of primary treatment (oxytocin/ergometrine) (See Chapter 9 on Obstetric Haemorrhage, and PPH flow chart in Appendix 2).
- It is given as an intramuscular injection of 250 µg and can be repeated at intervals of not less than 15 minutes to a maximum of 8 doses.
- Side effects include bronchospasm, pulmonary oedema and hypertension and so it should be used with caution in asthmatics. It may also cause transient pyrexia due to its effect on hypothalamic thermoregulation.

> Carboprost 250 µg IM may be used during Caesarean section if there is a failure of uterine contraction or for PPH.

Tocolytics

The main use for tocolytics is to stop premature labour. They have also been used to facilitate delivery during Caesarean section by uterine relaxation and to treat uterine hyperstimulation, preventing fetal distress.

In the treatment of premature labour, ritodrine is no longer the drug of choice, alternatives such as atosiban or nifedipine appear to have comparable effectiveness with fewer maternal side effects.

Atosiban

- Oxytocin antagonist.
- Used to arrest premature or threatened labour.
- Better tolerated than beta-agonists, atosiban appears to be highly specific with minimal side effects.
- Acts by competing with oxytocin at the receptor level on the myometrial plasma membrane, and may also prevent oxytocin-mediated release of prostaglandins.[6]
- An initial intravenous bolus dose of 6.75 mg is given over a minute, followed by a continuous infusion of 300 μg/min for 3 hours. This is then decreased to 100 μg/min for up to a maximum of 45 hours. Total maximum length of treatment is 48 hours to a maximum dose of 330 mg.

Nifedipine

- Calcium channel blocker, which reduces calcium influx into cells, reducing muscle contractility.
- A 2002 meta-analysis reviewed 12 RCTs and found that nifedipine is more effective than ritodrine and much safer. There is also evidence of improved neonatal outcomes.[7]
- A variety of dose regimes have been tested. The protocol from the largest trial is 10 mg orally stat, followed by 10 mg orally every 15 minutes for 1 hour if contractions persist, followed by 60–160 mg orally in split doses for 48–72 hours.
- Prolonged maintenance for tocolysis therapy is not recommended at present.[8,9]
- Contraindications include hepatic dysfunction, significant maternal cardiac disease and allergy to nifedipine.
- Reported side effects are hypotension, palpitations, flushing, headache and nausea.
- At present not licensed for tocolysis in the UK.

Beta$_2$-adrenergic agonists

- No longer used to suppress premature labour due to side effects (tachycardia and hypotension).
- Nebulised or inhaled **salbutamol** has been used to facilitate fetal delivery during Caesarean section.
- **Terbutaline**, 250 μg sc is the drug recommended by NICE for tocolysis during IOL in the presence of uterine hypercontractility and an abnormal fetal heat rate.[1]

Magnesium

- Better known for the prevention and treatment of seizures but is also an effective tocolytic. Used in the USA and other parts of the world, but rarely in the UK.

Glyceryl trinitrate

- Has been used to provide rapid uterine relaxation to facilitate vaginal and operative delivery. Efficacy and optimal dosing have not yet been established.
- Routes and doses used have included sublingual (800 µg) and IV (50–500 µg).

Volatile anaesthetic agents

- Decrease uterine muscle tone when their blood concentrations are greater than 0.5 MAC, but the oxytocic response is not lost until levels are greater than 0.9 MAC. This technique is useful when there is increased tone obstructing delivery by Caesarean section or for delivery of retained placenta, when general anaesthesia is used.
- The reduction in uterine tone does increase the likelihood of bleeding after delivery.

Anti-D

Since the introduction of postnatal Anti-D immunoprophylaxis in 1969, the incidence of haemolytic disease of the newborn (HDN) has plummeted to 1 in 21 000 births. However, even with meticulous immunoprophylaxis after delivery, immunisation still occurs in 1% of British mothers due to small feto-maternal haemorrhages that occur during pregnancy.

Studies show that antenatal prophylaxis (at 28/40 and 34/40) could reduce sensitisation to less than 0.1%. Therefore guidelines have been published by the RCOG and NICE concerning both antenatal and postnatal prophylaxis.[10,11]

Antenatal: It is recommended that 100 µg (500 IU) anti-D is given to all Rhesus-negative non-sensitised pregnant women at 28 and 34 weeks' gestation.

Postnatal: 100 µg (500 IU) anti-D immunoglobulin as soon as possible after delivery (certainly within 72 hours). A Kleihauer test is also performed to identify women with a large feto-maternal haemorrhage who would need additional immunoglobulin. Anti-D is given as a deep IM injection and may rarely cause an allergic reaction.

Magnesium

- Indications – the prevention of seizures in severe pre-eclampsia and management of eclamptic seizures.
- The Magpie trial (2002), compared magnesium sulphate with placebo for women with pre-eclampsia. It more than halved the risk of eclampsia and probably reduced the risk of maternal death. There did not appear to be any harmful effects on the baby.[12]
- Mode of action is not fully understood but is thought to behave as a calcium antagonist and to be involved with the uptake, binding and distribution of calcium in smooth muscle cells. It is also a potent cerebral vasodilator.

- It is presented as 50% magnesium sulphate in 10 ml ampoules, each containing 5 g (20 mmol).
- It is given as a loading dose of 4 g over 5–10 minutes followed by a maintenance infusion of 1 g/hr. Magnesium toxicity is unlikely with this regime and can be assessed effectively by monitoring deep tendon reflexes, respiratory rate and urine output as clinical effects are directly related to plasma levels (see Table 13.1).
- Side effects include flushing, nasal stuffiness, headache and hypotension.

Magnesium regime (example):
- Loading dose, 4 g (made up to 40 ml infused at 240 ml/hr)
- Maintenance, 1–2 g/hr, (given as 5 g made up to 50 ml infused at 10–20 ml/hr)

Antihypertensives

Antihypertensive agents are widely used in pregnancy but they all cross the placenta and the available evidence does not always suggest that they are of benefit.

Mild and pre-existing hypertension
- Two Cochrane reviews found that antihypertensives may halve the risk of severe hypertension but show no clear effect on other important outcomes such as pre-eclampsia or perinatal death. They conclude that it remains unclear whether any significant benefit is achieved by treating mild to moderate hypertension in pregnancy with medication.[13,14]
- If the woman is not taking any antihypertensive treatment, close monitoring without treatment may be appropriate.
- Drugs used most often are oral methyldopa, labetalol and nifedipine. The mode of action and side effects and further comments are shown in Table 13.2.

Table 13.1 Magnesium: clinical effects and plasma levels

	Plasma levels (mmol/l)
Therapeutic levels	2.0– 4.0
ECG Changes (wide QRS, prolonged PR)	3.0–5.0
Loss of deep tendon reflexes	>5.0
Heart block, CNS and respiratory depression	>7.5
Cardiac arrest	>12

Table 13.2 Antihypertensives commonly used in pregnancy

Drug	Type	Comment
Methyldopa	Centrally acting	Has been used extensively without reports of short or long term adverse effects on the fetus
		No effect on uteroplacental or renal blood flow, fetal haemodynamics or maternal cardiac output
Labetalol	Beta-blocker	Extensively used without reports of adverse effects on the fetus. Other β-blockers seldom used due to limited safety data. Should be avoided in asthmatics
Hydralazine	Vasodilator	Appears to be safe although a few cases of fetal thrombocytopenia have been reported
		Normally restricted to IV use in hypertensive emergencies
		Poorly tolerated orally due to side effects such as palpitations, headache and dizziness
Nifedipine	Calcium-channel blocker	No evidence of harm to the fetus but limited safety data
		Modified-release preparation recommended in preference to standard-release product, which may cause a precipitous drop in blood pressure

Acute management of severe hypertension

- Treatment is recommended for severe hypertension. Guidelines usually recommend antihypertensive treatment if the systolic blood pressure exceeds 160 mmHg or if the diastolic pressure exceeds 110 mmHg.[15]
- Oral/IV labetalol, oral nifedipine and IV hydralazine are used in the acute management of severe hypertension.
- Avoid atenolol, ACE inhibitors, angiotensin receptor antagonists and diuretics in pregnancy.

Currently there is insufficient evidence to recommend one antihypertensive in preference to another and so the choice of which to use is likely to depend on personal preference and availability.

Antihypertensive regimes (examples)

Hydralazine:
- 10–20 mg IV given over 20 minutes to a maximum cumulative dose of 20 mg
- followed by an infusion of 40 mg in 40 ml of normal saline running at 1–10 ml/hr.

Labetalol:
- 50 mg IV given over 10 minutes
- followed by an infusion of labetalol solution at 20–160 mg/hr.

Steroids

There is good evidence that a single course of steroids reduces neonatal mortality, lowers the incidence and severity of intraventricular haemorrhage and necrotising enterocolitis, and halves respiratory morbidity when there is the threat of delivery to a fetus of 24–34 weeks' gestation.[16] Indications include:

- Threatened preterm labour
- Antepartum haemorrhage
- Preterm rupture of membranes
- Conditions necessitating elective preterm delivery

Delivery should be delayed by a minimum of 12 hours to observe the benefits of antenatal steroids, and these benefits are proven to last for 7 days.

Recommended regimes include **Betamethasone** 12 mg IM every 12 hours for 2 doses, or **Dexamethasone** 6 mg IM every 6 hours for 4 doses.[16]

The benefit of repeated courses of steroids has not been proven;[17] rather, multivariate analyses have shown that increasing the number of antenatal exposure of steroids is associated with reduced cognitive function, an increase in behavioural disorders and reduced birth weight.[18] There may also be deleterious effects on the hypothalamo–pituitary axis and glucose homeostasis.

REFERENCES

1. National Institute for Health and Clinical Excellence. *Inherited Clinical Guideline D. Induction of Labour* (London: Department of Health, 2001).
2. A. Gülmezoglu, F. Forna, J. Villar and G. Hofmeyr, Prostaglandins for preventing postpartum haemorrhage. *Cochrane Database Syst. Rev.*, 3 (2007), CD000494. DOI 10.1002/14651858.CD000494.pub2.
3. C. Langenbach, Misoprostol in preventing postpartum haemorrhage: a meta-analysis. *Int. J. Gynecol. Obstet.*, **92** (2006), 10–18.
4. P. O'Brien, H. El-Refaey, A. Gordon, M. Geary and C. H. Rodeck, Rectally administered misoprostol for the treatment of postpartum hemorrhage unresponsive to oxytocin and ergometrine: a descriptive study. *Obstet. Gynecol*, **92**:2 (1998), 212–4.
5. A. U. Lokugamage, K. R. Sullivan, I. Niculescu *et al*. A randomized study comparing rectally administered misoprostol versus Syntometrine combined with an oxytocin infusion for the cessation of primary postpartum haemorrhage. *Acta Obstet. Gynecol. Scand.*, **80**:9 (2001), 835–9.
6. P. Melin, Oxytocin antagonists in preterm labour and delivery. *Bailliere's Clin. Obstet. Gynaecol.*, **7** (1993), 577–600.
7. V. Tsatsaris, D. Patapsonis, F. Goffinet, G. Dekker and B. Carbonne, Tocolysis with nifedipine or beta-adrenergic agonists: a meta-analysis. *Obstet. Gynecol.* **97** (2001), 840–7.

8. N. Gaunekar and C. A. Crowther, Maintenance therapy with calcium channel blockers for preventing preterm birth after threatened preterm labour. *Cochrane Database Syst. Rev.*, **3** (2004), CD004071. DOI 10.1002/14651858.CD004071.pub2.

9. Royal College of Obstetricians and Gynaecologists, *Tocolytic Drugs for Women in Preterm Labour*. Guideline Number 1B (London: RCOG Press, 2002).

10. Royal College of Obstetricians and Gynaecologists, *Anti-D Immunoglobulin for Rhesus Prophylaxis*. Guideline Number 22 (London: RCOG Press, 2002).

11. National Institute for Health and Clinical Excellence, *The Use of Routine Antenatal Anti-D Prophylaxis for Rhesus-D Negative Women*. Technology Appraisal Guidance number 41 (London: Department of Health, 2002).

12. The Magpie Trial Collaboration Group. Do women with pre-eclampsia, and their babies, benefit from magnesium sulphate? The Magpie Trial: a randomised placebo-controlled trial. *Lancet*, **359** (2002), 1877–90.

13. E. Abalos, L. Duley, D. W. Steyn and D. J. Henderson-Smart, Anti-hypertensive drug therapy for mild–moderate hypertension during pregnancy. *Cochrane Database Syst. Rev.*, **1** (2007), CD002252. DOI 10.1002/14651858.CD002252.pub2.

14. L. A. Magee and L. Duley, Oral beta-blockers for mild to moderate hypertension during pregnancy. *Cochrane Database Syst. Rev.*, **1** (2003), CD002863. DOI 10.1002/14651858.CD002863.pub2.

15. L. Duley, D. J. Henderson-Smart and S. Meher, Drugs for treatment of very high blood pressure during pregnancy. *Cochrane Database Syst. Rev.*, **3** (2006), CD001449. DOI 10.1002/14651858. CD001449.pub2.

16. Royal College of Obstetricians and Gynaecologists, *Antenatal Corticosteroids to Prevent Respiratory Distress Syndrome*. Guideline Number 7 (London: RCOG Press, 2004).

17. D. A. Guinn, M. W. Atkinson, L. Sullivan *et al.*, Single vs weekly courses of antenatal corticosteroids for women at risk of preterm labour: a randomised controlled trial. *JAMA*, **286**:13 (2001), 1581–7.

18. H. H. Kay, I. M. Bird, C. L. Coe and D. J. Dudley, Antenatal steroid treatment and adverse fetal effects: what is the evidence? *J. Soc. Gynecol. Investig.*, **7**:5 (2000), 269–78.

FURTHER READING

K. G. Eagland and G. M. Cooper, Drugs acting on the uterus. *Bulletin 10 The Royal College of Anaesthetists November 2001*, 473–6.

J. M. Roberts, Preventing and treating eclamptic seizures. *BMJ*, **325** (2002), 609–10.

L. Duley and J. P. Neilson, Magnesium sulphate and pre-eclampsia. *BMJ*, **319** (1999), 3–4.

Confidential enquiries into fetal, neonatal and maternal death

Katie Clift

Introduction

Until April 2003 there were two separate bodies collecting information and making enquiries into maternal and perinatal deaths in the UK. The Confidential Enquiries into Maternal Deaths (CEMD) produced triennial reports entitled "Why Mothers Die" from 1952 up to and including the report for 1997/9. The Confidential Enquiries into Stillbirths and Deaths in Infancy (CESDI) produced annual reports in addition to focused reports (e.g. Project 27/28).

These two bodies are now combined into the Confidential Enquiry into Maternal and Child Health (CEMACH). This is a self-governing body managed by its own board with members nominated by eight Royal Colleges. The remit of CEMACH includes the improvement of maternal and child health as well as mortality reviews. To this end, CEMACH has not only continued the Why Mothers Die report and the Stillbirth Neonatal and Postnatal Mortality report but also undertakes focused enquiries e.g. The Diabetes Study.

The National Institute for Health and Clinical Excellence (NICE) currently takes overall responsibility for the publishing of these reports, however this role will be short lived and is soon to be handed over to the National Patient Safety Agency (NPSA).

All maternal deaths should be reported to CEMACH Regional Manager, who then initiates an enquiry by sending a standard form to all professionals concerned with the care of the woman. The Trust must hold an internal investigation to ascertain what happened, and the Strategic Health Authorities, Primary Care Trust, coroner, and Local Supervising Authority Midwifery Officer (LSAMO) should also be informed.

Maternal death – main causes

Definitions

Direct deaths Deaths resulting from obstetric complications of the pregnant state (pregnancy, labour and puerperium), from interventions, omissions, incorrect treatment or from a chain of events resulting from any of the above.

Indirect deaths Deaths resulting from previous existing disease, or disease that developed during pregnancy and which was not due to direct obstetric causes, but which was aggravated by the physiologic effects of pregnancy.

Internationally, 80% of maternal deaths are due to direct causes and 20% due to indirect causes. In contrast, the last two triennial reports have recorded more indirect than direct deaths.

Obstetrics for Anaesthetists, ed. Alexander Heazell and John Clift. Published by Cambridge University Press. © Cambridge University Press 2008

Table 14.1. Main causes of direct maternal death in the UK

	No of deaths in 2000–2
Thrombosis and thromboembolism	30
Haemorrhage	17
Early pregnancy deaths	15
Hypertensive disease of pregnancy	14
Genital tract sepsis	11
Anaesthetic deaths	6
Amniotic fluid embolism	5

The main causes of *direct* maternal deaths in the UK are shown in Table 14.1.

The *direct* maternal mortality rate for the triennium 2000–2 was 5.3 deaths per 100 000 maternities. This was higher than the immediately preceding triennium but lower than the three preceding that.

The only *direct* cause of maternal mortality to rise in the most recently reported triennium was haemorrhage. On closer examination of the causes, the number of deaths due to placental abruption and placental praevia were unchanged, but the death-rate due to postpartum haemorrhage increased tenfold.

The reasons for this rise are not clear, and probably multiple. However the anaesthetists' role in resuscitation is paramount and the recommendations from this report reflect this.

The major causes of *indirect* maternal deaths reported in the last triennium were cardiac, psychiatric and malignancies. Of particular significance is the proportion of psychiatric deaths due to suicide, especially when the late deaths (up to one year) are included. The CEMACH has now introduced Regional Psychiatric Assessors to facilitate a more detailed assessment of this for the next "Why Mothers Die" report.

Fetal and neonatal death – main causes

Definitions

Stillbirth A child that has issued forth from its mother after the 24th week of pregnancy and who did not at any time after being completely expelled from its mother breathe or show any other signs of life.

Early neonatal death Death of a live born baby occurring less than 7 completed days from the time of birth.

Late neonatal death Death of a live born baby occurring from the 7th day of life and before 28 completed days from the time of birth.

The main causes of stillbirths reported in the CEMACH Perinatal Mortality Surveillance 2004 were:

Unexplained antepartum fetal death	50.6%
Congenital anomaly	15.1%
Antepartum haemorrhage	10.0%
Death from intrapartum causes	7.3%
Pre-eclampsia	3.5%

The main causes of early and late neonatal deaths in the same report were:

Immaturity	48.0%
Congenital anomaly	22.4%
Death from intrapartum causes	10.9%
Infection	6.8%
Sudden infant death	2.5%

The stillbirth rate increased significantly between 2001 and 2002 (5.4 to 5.7 per 1000 births and this rise has been sustained. The CEMACH is conducting a trend analysis of the risk factors associated with stillbirths between 1994–2004 in response to this. The neonatal mortality rate in 2004 was 3.4 per 1000 births, which represents a decreasing trend. Both stillbirth and neonatal mortality rates are higher in women in socially deprived areas and in women of Black or Asian ethnicity. Multiple births have higher stillbirth and neonatal mortality rates.

Anaesthesia and maternal death

Each CEMACH report generates a series of recommendations for clinical practice and service provision. The recommendations for anaesthesia services from the most recent "Why Mothers Die" (2000–2002) report are summarised below:

There were a total of seven deaths felt to be attributable to anaesthesia, although there were frequently other contributory factors. Of note, one third of all the maternal deaths were women who were obese, and this has lead to the recommendation that pregnant women with a body mass index greater than 35 be referred early to the anaesthetic service to establish a management plan.

The failure to recognise oesophageal intubation resulted in three deaths during this triennium (one of these was an anaesthetic given for ruptured ectopic pregnancy). In all three cases the mistake was made by a Senior House Officer grade anaesthetist without immediate senior back-up. The emphasis is back on airway training and the level of training of frontline anaesthetists.

The number of high-risk cases, especially women with cardiac disease, is increasing. When required, obstetric anaesthetists should not hesitate to call on the assistance of anaesthetic colleagues in other subspecialities and colleagues in other disciplines. Cases at high risk of or with major haemorrhage should involve a consultant obstetric anaesthetist at the earliest possible time. Invasive monitoring is recommended when the cardiovascular system is compromised. Arterial blood gas analysis should be obtained early and metabolic acidosis taken seriously. Early commencement of intensive therapy must be instituted and consultant-to-consultant referral is recommended.

Anaesthetists, and colleagues in other relevant disciplines, should be involved in the care of high-risk patients from early in pregnancy and a management plan made for the care of these women

FURTHER INFORMATION

www.cemach.org.uk – website of Confidential Enquiry into Maternal and Child Health.

Adult Advanced Life Support Algorithm

Adult Advanced Life Support Algorithm

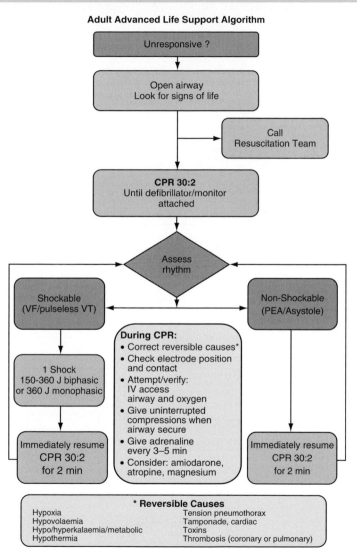

Left Lateral tilt: Consider Perimortem Caesarean Section if ≥ 24 weeks gestation

If on IV Magnesium Sulphate give 10 ml 10% Calcium Gluconate

The Management of Postpartum Haemorrhage Algorithm

The Management of Postpartum Haemorrhage Algorithm

Initial assessment and treatment			
Communication:	**Resuscitation:**	**Assess Aetiology:**	**Laboratory Tests:**
Explain and reassure patient Call experienced midwife Call obstetric registrar and alert consultant Call anaesthetic registrar and alert consultant Alert blood transfusion service Call porters	ABC High flow O_2 Tilt head down, avoid supine 2×14G cannulae \Rapid fluid replacement Monitor vital signs, SaO_2 and ECG Insert Foley catheter and monitor urine output	Abdominal assessment of uterine tone and tissue Explore lower genital tract Exclude ruptured or inverted uterus	FBC Clotting ABO blood grouping and X match 6 units

Once 3.5 litres of clear fluid (colloid or crystalloid) are given blood should be transfused:
1. X matched (if available)
2. Group specific
3. "O neg"(if others not available)

Treat the cause (4 Ts)			
Tone:	**Tissue:**	**Trauma:**	**Thrombin:**
Uterine massage Oxytocin 10 U slow IV Ergometrine 0.5 mg slow IV Oxytocin infusion 10 U/hr Carboprost 250 µg IM (rpt >15 min, max. 5 doses)	Remove retained products	Direct pressure Repair/suture Manual or hydrostatic replacement of inverted uterus under anaesthesia	Correction of clotting abnormalities

Intractable PPH		
Get help:	**Local control:**	**BP and coagulation:**
2nd experienced surgeon 2nd experienced anaesthetist Haematologist Critical Care Staff	Bimanual compression Pack uterus/vagina	Fluid replacement using fluid warming device Blood products Invasive monitoring FBC, U&Es, clotting, blood gases

Surgery
Direct intramyometrial injection Carboprost 250 µg at laparotomy Bilateral uterine artery embolisation/ligation Bilateral internal iliac artery ligation B-lynch suture Hysterectomy

Post-Hysterectomy Bleeding
Abdominal packing Angiographic embolisation Correction of coagulopathy Admit to Critical Care Unit

Emergency Management of Eclamptic Fit Algorithm

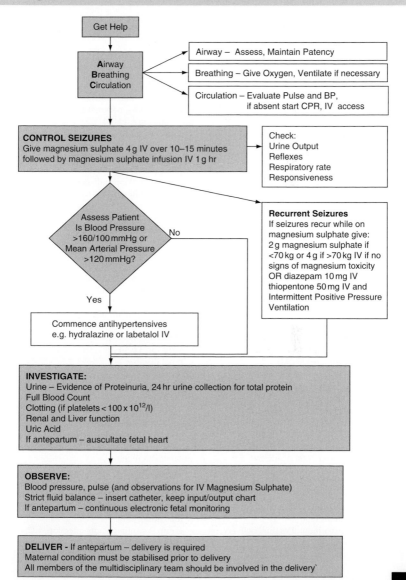

Get Help

Airway **B**reathing **C**irculation

Airway – Assess, Maintain Patency

Breathing – Give Oxygen, Ventilate if necessary

Circulation – Evaluate Pulse and BP,
if absent start CPR, IV access

CONTROL SEIZURES
Give magnesium sulphate 4 g IV over 10–15 minutes
followed by magnesium sulphate infusion IV 1 g hr

Check:
Urine Output
Reflexes
Respiratory rate
Responsiveness

Assess Patient
Is Blood Pressure
>160/100 mmHg or
Mean Arterial Pressure
>120 mmHg?

No

Recurrent Seizures
If seizures recur while on
magnesium sulphate give:
2 g magnesium sulphate if
<70 kg or 4 g if >70 kg IV if no
signs of magnesium toxicity
OR diazepam 10 mg IV
thiopentone 50 mg IV and
Intermittent Positive Pressure
Ventilation

Yes

Commence antihypertensives
e.g. hydralazine or labetalol IV

INVESTIGATE:
Urine – Evidence of Proteinuria, 24 hr urine collection for total protein
Full Blood Count
Clotting (if platelets < 100 x 10^{12}/l)
Renal and Liver function
Uric Acid
If antepartum – auscultate fetal heart

OBSERVE:
Blood pressure, pulse (and observations for IV Magnesium Sulphate)
Strict fluid balance – insert catheter, keep input/output chart
If antepartum – continuous electronic fetal monitoring

DELIVER - If antepartum – delivery is required
Maternal condition must be stabilised prior to delivery
All members of the multidisciplinary team should be involved in the delivery`

Index